1001
BEAUTY
SOLUTIONS

Beth Barrick-Hickey

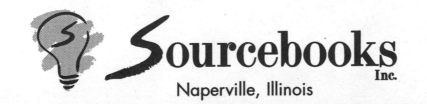

Sourcebooks
Inc.
Naperville, Illinois

Published by: **Sourcebooks, Inc.**
P.O. Box 372, Naperville, Illinois, 60566
(708) 961-3900
FAX: 708-961-2168

This publication is designed to provide accurate and authoritative information in regard to the subject matter covered. It is sold with the understanding that the publisher is not engaged in rendering legal, accounting, or other professional service. If legal advice or other expert assistance is required, the services of a competent professional person should be sought.

From a Declaration of Principles Jointly Adopted by a Committee of the
American Bar Association and a Committee of Publishers and Associations

Library of Congress Cataloging-in-Publication Data
Barrick-Hickey, Beth
        1001 beauty solutions : the ultimate one-step adviser for your everyday beauty problems / by Beth Barrick-Hickey.
            p.   cm.
        ISBN 1-57071-049-X
        1. Beauty, Personal.   2. Hair—Care and hygiene.   3. Skin—Care and hygiene.   4. Cosmetics.   I. Title.
    RA778.B2343   1995
    646.7'2 — dc20   95-24937
                                                                                                 CIP

Printed and bound in the United States of America.

10   9   8   7   6   5   4   3   2   1

Contents

Acknowledgments

When my first book "500 Beauty Solutions" came out, who would have thought that it would have stirred so many women to respond with questions and comments about their most common beauty concerns? Thanks to the overwhelming response of women as well as MEN to "500 Beauty Solutions," it became apparent that a more comprehensive guide to hair, skin and nails was needed. "1001 Beauty Solutions" updates the information in "500 Beauty Solutions" and provides new information on hair care, skin care, makeup and depilatory procedures, all in an easy-to-read, question-and-answer format.

What makes "1001 Beauty Solutions" truly unique is the professional perspective from which it is written. Salon owners, stylists, research and development experts, nail technicians, estheticians, beauty marketing professionals as well as beauty editors, and the merchandising staff of Sally Beauty Supply all contributed to this comprehensive beauty guide.

Credit belongs to my colleague, Susan Walker, vice president of marketing for Sally Beauty Supply, who gathered together her store managers, merchandising staff, and vendors representing the top names in beauty to collect hundreds of professional answers to these beauty questions.

We consulted Dr. Diane L. Gibby, founder of the Women's Center for Plastic and Reconstructive Surgery at Medical City in Dallas, for the latest information on skin care, including alpha hydroxy acids and Retin-A.

For our hair care chapters, we sought the advice of Dayton Mast, owner of L'Image Salons and a member of Intercoiffure International, as well as one of his top stylists, Stephen Minton, and nail technician, Jamie Harry. Additional aromatherapy information was provided by Gio Punto of Capelli Punto Salon in New York. Expert makeup application tips and techniques were generously supplied by New York makeup artist Ilise Heitzner Harris.

Hundreds of questions as well as answers were provided by the professional hair care divisions of Clairol, L'Oreal, Revlon, Wella, Helene Curtis, Conair, Zotos and Summit Laboratories.

"1001 Beauty Solutions" would not have been possible without the research assistance provided by Leanne Lalor, Jane Anne McPhee, and Catherine Person in Dallas, and Katharine Bernard in New York for her skin care and makeup research. For the arduous process of organizing all the data, cross-referencing and preparation of the manuscript, thanks go to Suzanne Schaffler in Dallas of The Hart Agency. I am grateful for the creative direction and lighthearted, easy-to-read design of the book provided by graphic designer Bill Ford of Ford and Company. Drawings were contributed by artist Sheilah James in New York.

A final note of thanks to beauty and marketing specialists, Jane Gyulavary in New York and Rosanne Hart in Dallas, who conceived the book and worked closely with me in its development.

It is our hope that this newly revised version of "500 Beauty Solutions," entitled "1001 Beauty Solutions," answers all of your most common beauty concerns in a clear, conversational manner that not only saves you time but also money. Think of the book as your own beauty expert—always on call 'round the clock between salon visits!

—Beth Barrick-Hickey

Thank you to my husband, Emmett, and to my family for their support and enthusiasm throughout this project.
—Beth

Introduction

Long before the days of Cleopatra, women regarded hair as their crowning glory. Beauty regimens have a history as old as time itself. And if there is one thing that has held true throughout the ages, it is that women have always sought ways to improve the way they look.

As we edge closer to the 21st century, more and more products fill the shelves of drug stores, grocery chains, salons and beauty supply outlets. The endless array is mind-boggling, overwhelming and confusing at best! What shampoo should you use? What brush won't split ends? Which nail file works best on acrylic nails? What are AHAs? How do I make my eyes look bigger?

Colorful labels, beautifully illustrated packaging, bold claims, sweepstakes and two-for-one promotions beckon us at every turn as we search for just the right beauty solution.

"1001 Beauty Solutions" adds 501 new questions and answers to the original beauty guide, "500 Beauty Solutions," and includes an expanded chapter on ethnic hair care, as well as two new chapters for skin care and makeup application. Over 150 pages, this comprehensive beauty guide is designed to help you cut through the clutter to solve your most common hair, nail, skin and makeup concerns. You may have wanted to ask these same questions of your stylist. And when you have a beauty crisis that erupts at the most inopportune time, "1001 Beauty Solutions" will come to the rescue.

Straight talk is all there is. No weighty technical jargon that requires a chemistry degree. No heavy blocks of copy you have to wade through to find a solution. It's all here, in a simple, question-and-answer format, much like you might find in a magazine beauty column.

HOW TO USE THIS BOOK

"1001 Beauty Solutions" takes the guesswork out of what really works when it comes to solving a myriad of beauty problems and having healthy hair and nails.

You'll discover, however, not only how to solve a problem, but also what specifically to use—and how to use it! Who better than the professionals to give you advice on how to care for your hair, skin and nails?

Most of the products mentioned in this book are available through beauty salons, beauty supply stores or the more than 1,500 Sally Beauty Supply stores throughout the world. Many of the products mentioned are comparable to branded lines available only in salons. What makes the products mentioned in this book unique, in many cases, is that they offer not only professional quality, but also value. And in these times of growing budgetary concerns, affordability is an important issue.

"1001 Beauty Solutions" is divided into 12 chapters, each almost equally devoted to advice and product-specific solutions. This newly revised version of "500 Beauty Solutions" includes extensive information on hair and nail care, as well as skin care and makeup. The chapter devoted to the needs of women of color has been expanded to include more up-to-date information and products related to hair color and relaxing.

Sprinkled throughout the chapters is FY👁, information that is basic to understanding how to properly care for hair, nails and skin.

As more and more consumers, as well as beauty media, looked to Sally Beauty Supply and other beauty professionals for the answers to their beauty questions, it became clear that a more complete beauty guide was needed that addressed the most common beauty concerns of women from a professional point of view.

For the millions of women who walk into a Sally Beauty Supply, a drug store, beauty salon or department store to purchase their beauty products, the question often arises, "There's so much here, where do I begin?"

Start here, with your very first question. Then keep it handy when a beauty question comes up. Stash it in your bathroom vanity drawer. Take it with you on vacation, or when you travel on business. Whatever you do, don't leave home without it! You never know when a 911 beauty emergency will strike!

CHAPTER ONE

Shampoo To Maintain Your Mane

The word "shampoo" was born in England when British hairdressers coined the word "shampoo" from the Hindu word "champo" which means "to massage" or "to knead." But it was not until the 1890s in Germany that the first actual detergent-based shampoo was introduced to the world. Previously, cleansing solutions for the hair were concocted as early as ancient Egyptian times when the Egyptians mixed water and citrus juice to remove the hair's sebum oil.

The modern shampoo business owes its beginning in America to John Breck who developed various hair and scalp cleansing solutions in hopes of curing his early-onset baldness. Breck first came up with shampoos for normal hair which were popular in beauty salons in the '30s. Later, he developed a complete shampoo line for oily and dry hair. Although he had built an empire of hair care products, Breck was not able to stop his own baldness.

Today, there are hundreds of shampoos available, from expensive brand names lining cosmetic counters of the finest department stores to promotionally priced gallons at your local discounter.

Shampoos do more than just clean hair and stimulate the scalp. In your salon, your stylist uses special formulations of shampoo to prepare hair for chemical services, such as perms or hair color. Shampoos are also helpful in adding body, texture and shine to hair. Some revive color, while others can strip away styling product build-up or even chlorine from the pool.

The key to selecting the right shampoo for you is the type of hair you have. Is it normal, oily, dry, fine, coarse or chemically treated? The condition of your hair is important, as well. When visiting your stylist, ask to have your hair analyzed. Your stylist can help you make the right choice.

F.Y.👁 The pH Factor

The term "pH" refers to the balance between acid and alkaline, which must be measured with the presence of water, because dry substances do not have a pH. pH ranges from 0 to 14, with 7.0 being neutral, like water. Anything under 7.0 is acid, anything above is alkaline. Human hair seems to like a mildly acid pH level. Although hair has no pH, the scalp and the natural oils which coat the cuticle of the hair do have a pH between 4.5 and 5.5. Shampoos that claim to be pH-balanced usually range from 4.5 to 6.5. Basically, pH-balanced means that the shampoo is gentle, not harsh.

1. Are professional shampoo products really different than those found in grocery, drug or department stores?

Yes! There are significant differences in professional shampoo products. Some contain higher concentrations of certain ingredients, such as protein. A key benefit is that salon or professional shampoos are often developed based on the hair stylist's actual experiences, rather than the manufacturers' marketing surveys! Professional shampoos have a pH of 4.5 to 6.5, and emollients and cleansers are blended to break dirt and oil into tiny particles that slide off hair and scalp harmlessly.

2. Is there a shampoo that will make my hair grow faster?

No shampoo will <u>grow</u> hair, but there are several that help add fullness and that clean well to keep scalp healthy, which aids in allowing hair to grow faster. John Breck spent much of his career trying to answer that same question. Try Folicure Shampoo, VazoCure Antioxidant Shampoo or Jheri Redding Professional Prescription Biotin Shampoo.

3. What is an "everyday" shampoo?

Although most shampoos are designed to be used every day, there are some products designated as "everyday" or "lighter formula" shampoos. These shampoos are usually milder and have a slightly acid pH level that hair likes. The most important thing to remember is to choose a shampoo that fits your hair type (normal, oily, dry, permed, colored). Acclaim Plus Daily Conditioning Shampoo, Ion Balanced Cleansing Shampoo, Quantum Shampoo, or Professional Prescription

Absolute Shampoo are considered "everyday" shampoos.

4. Is it necessary to shampoo my hair every day?

Frequency of shampooing varies with each individual, depending on lifestyle and the amount of oils secreted in the scalp. Always use a professional formula shampoo to keep hair healthy.

5. If I leave a shampoo on my hair for 2-3 minutes will it clean my hair better?

No. Shampoos are designed to attract soil and lift it off the hair. Shampoo does not absorb dirt.

TIP   Wash Cycle

Use a quarter-sized squeeze of shampoo. Lather the scalp first. After shampooing, always thoroughly rinse hair with cool water to prevent shampoo residue before conditioning.

---

6. Will frequent shampooing make my hair oilier?

No. Frequent shampooing will not make hair oilier, although excessive massage to the scalp will. Use an oily hair shampoo, such as Biotera Revitalizing Shampoo or a volume-building type, like Fermodyl Volumizing Shampoo.

7. I have so many different brands of shampoos in my bathroom. Should I use the same brand on my hair every day or should I alternate them?

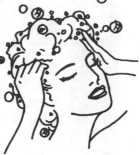

It's fine to use the same shampoo day after day, as long as you are using the correct shampoo for your hair type. Try using a clarifying shampoo periodically to eliminate any build-up.

8. Is it best to change shampoo brands often so my hair won't become immune to one kind?

Weather changes, rather than frequent use of one type or brand of shampoo, may prompt the need to change shampoos. In dry winter air, you may need a moisturizing shampoo, while summer may call for a volume-building shampoo that keeps hair looking fuller.

9. Should I use a regular bar soap to shampoo my hair every once in a while?

No. Bar soap is too alkaline and could strip hair color or perm and leave a fatty residue.

10. I love using styling products like mousse and gel to give my hair body, but I don't think my shampoo is getting rid of all that build-up. What should I do?

Use a gentle, deep cleansing shampoo routinely, once or twice a week. Depending on the build-up, use a deep cleanser or clarifying shampoo. A clarifying shampoo, which contains more detergent than an everyday shampoo, is designed to lightly strip the hair. It usually has a higher pH level, too. Use only as needed and follow with a conditioner. Try Quantum or Ion Clarifying Shampoo, Salon Care Ultra Moisturizing Anti-Chlorine Shampoo, Queen Helene RX-18 or Action Environmental Hard or Extra Hard Water Shampoo. Use once a week, but not more than twice a week.

11. What ingredients should I look for in a shampoo that will banish build-up?

Sodium laureth sulfate, which is a surfactant, adds cleansing properties to the shampoo—most shampoos have it. Avoid heavy conditioning shampoos which could add to the build-up problem. Good choices: Ion Clarifying Shampoo, Ion Balanced Cleansing Shampoo, Tresemme 4+4 Deep Cleansing Shampoo or Fantasia's 100% Pure Tea Shampoo.

12. What shampoo should I use that will get rid of the mineral build-up caused by hard water?

A clarifying shampoo used periodically should help. Salon Care Ultra Moisturizing Anti-Chlorine Shampoo, Action Environmental Hard Water or Extra Hard Water Shampoo or Avec's All Pure Purifying Shampoo work well on all mineral deposits.

13. I have heard that rusty water turns your hair a reddish tint. Is this true?

Yes. Chemicals in water can discolor porous hair resulting in orange or brownish stains.

Try Action Environmental Hard Water or Extra Hard Water Shampoo to eliminate this problem.

14. What shampoo do I use to get rid of medication build-up on my hair?

Use a good clarifying shampoo like Ion Clarifying Shampoo or Avec's All Pure Shampoo. You may also want to check with your doctor.

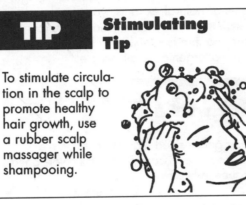

TIP **Stimulating Tip**

To stimulate circulation in the scalp to promote healthy hair growth, use a rubber scalp massager while shampooing.

15. What makes a body-building shampoo work?

It cleanses without leaving any residual conditioner on hair. It has a rinse-clean factor to make hair feel fuller by leaving the hair cuticle slightly ruffled. Try Ion Balanced Cleansing, Jheri Redding Volumizer, Revlon Fermodyl Volumizing Shampoo or Biotera Revitalizing shampoos.

16. My hair is straight, fine and very thin. Is there a particular shampoo that will give my hair body and fullness?

Try a volumizing formula, like Volumax, Jheri

Redding Volumizer, Folicure or Acclaim Daily Conditioning Shampoo. The key ingredient is panthenol (Vitamin B-5) which acts to "plump up" the hair shaft.

17. What are the benefits of natural sources, such as botanicals, eggs, honey, aloe vera, etc., in shampoo?

Natural source botanicals add proteins and conditioning agents to shampoo. They may be derived from plant and vegetable extracts or other sources. The benefit to hair is that they contain proteins and moisture in a natural state, and could be an alternative for those with a sensitive scalp. Biotera, Mixx Essential Sudz, Jheri Redding Professional Prescription Transpose and Aura shampoos contain natural extracts.

18. I like to use botanical products on my hair. Do they clean my hair as well as other types of shampoos?

Many do clean just as well, as they usually contain a detergent which is needed for cleansing. Pure botanical extracts from flowers and plant oils can be found in Aura shampoos, Aphogee Evening Primrose Moisture Shampoo and Mixx Essential Sudz. All are mildly refreshing, yet thoroughly cleanse hair.

19. What do herbs do for my hair?

Spearmint acts as an antiseptic that helps clean an oily scalp. Camomile is believed to

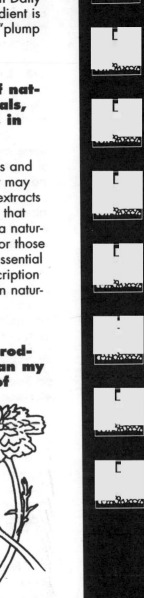

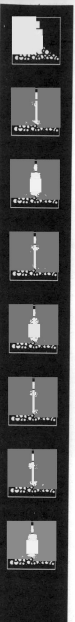

lighten hair. Comfrey and rosemary aid in cleansing. Try Aura shampoos, specially formulated with herbs and botanicals.

20. I would like to enhance my own natural hair color. What highlighting shampoos are available, and what do they do?

These shampoos have color added in the form of vegetable dyes that tone the hair. They are made to highlight or add depth to hair color, or provide a specific shading effect. Read the labels to find out what hair color the shampoo will enhance, for example, Aura Shampoo with Madder Root for redheads, Clove for brunettes, Camomile for blondes, Black Malva for black hair, L'Oreal Programme Colour in beige, gold, copper, mahogany and chestnut; and Clairol's Shimmer Lights Gold Formula to add gold to blonde hair.

21. I have gray hair which tends to look dingy. How do I take the yellow out?

You need to use a highlighting shampoo which contains vegetable dyes that tone down hair. These shampoos can minimize that brassy, yellow look with a gentle cool blue or violet base color. Try using Clairol's Shimmer Lights Original Formula or Jheri Redding Silver Lustre.

22. My gray hair turned blue when I used a highlighting shampoo. What went wrong, and what can I use to keep it from looking brassy?

Gray hair can have many different textures and porosities which react differently to the amount of coloring found in color-enhancing shampoo. This is more of a problem with shampoos for toning brassiness on blonde hair, than for gray. Jheri Redding Silver Lustre and Aura Blue Malva have less blueing and are less likely to turn hair blue.

23. Because I am allergic to detergents, what is a quality hypo-allergenic shampoo?

Look for a shampoo with natural ingredients, such as Aura or Biotera. If you are allergic to plants or natural extracts, you may have an allergic reaction. There is no professional shampoo that is specifically hypo-allergenic or non-allergenic for all people.

TIP   **Bubble Bargain**

Buy gallon-sized jugs of your favorite shampoo and conditioner. Fill color-coded squeeze bottles—one for shampoo; one for conditioner—for easy use. Great for teens and back-to-college.

---

24. What shampoo is best for color-treated hair?

Shampoos that are designed to control color loss are lower in pH, ranging from 2.5 to 4, which forces the cuticle of the hair to close, thus enabling the hair to retain its color. Try Quantum Shampoo for Permed and Color-Treated Hair, Keragenics Rejuvenating Shampoo or L'Oreal Programme Colour Revitalizing Shampoo.

25. Can color-enhancing shampoos help maintain highlights, whether from color added to the hair or the sun's natural highlights?

Yes. Color-enhancing shampoos come in a variety of shades to complement all hair colors. Try Clairol Complements, L'Oreal Programme Colour or Aura.

26. My hair is really fried from perming. What type of shampoo will bring it back to life?

Normalizing shampoos take conditioning one step further. They are designed to revitalize hair dried out by chemical processes like perming. Sometimes they are called "perm rejuvenating" shampoos. Select a shampoo for permed hair, such as Quantum Shampoo for Permed and Color-Treated Hair, Professional Prescription Transpose, For Perms Only Original or Moisturizing shampoos or Ion Moisturizing Shampoo.

27. What shampoo should I use that has a sunscreen to protect my color from fading?

Try Aura, L'Oreal Programme Colour and Biotera shampoos, as well as Professional Prescription shampoos which contain conditioners as well as sunscreens.

28. I have dry hair. What shampoo should I use?

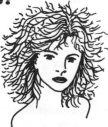

For dry hair, use a moisturizing shampoo which cleans and conditions. A moisturizing shampoo has a rinse-out conditioner mixed in to prevent loss of moisture by closing the cuticle, and it helps fight dryness caused by blow dryers, curling irons, heat rollers and sun. A good one to try is Ion Moisturizing Shampoo, Professional Prescription Transpose Shampoo, LaMaur Apple Pectin Moisturizing Shampoo, or Volumizer Moisturizing Shampoo with Extra Shine.

29. I get oily, greasy-looking hair at the end of the day. What can I do to end the greasies?

Use an oily-hair formula shampoo, such as Biotera Revitalizing Shampoo for Normal to Oily Hair, which can be used daily, or Quantum Clarifying Shampoo and Clarifying Shampoo from Ion, which should only be used twice a week. You may want to avoid using daily rinse-out conditioners, although you still need to condition hair. Fantasia IC 100% Pure Tea Shampoo also removes excess hair oils. Tea works as an astringent.

30. I have normal hair that has been chemically treated. What would be a gentle shampoo for me?

Use a daily shampoo with gentle cleansing properties, such as a moisturizing shampoo. Try Fermodyl Moisture Recovery, Keragenics Therapy or Aphogee Evening Primrose Oil Shampoo.

31. What is a good no-rinse shampoo that can be used when I can't take a shower or bath?

Try No-Rinse, a shampoo that you massage into your scalp and comb through. Let it dry. There is no need to rinse this shampoo out. It's great if you are bedridden or camping outdoors.

32. Will horse shampoos make my hair grow?

There is no shampoo product available that will make hair grow.

33. Can horse shampoos be used on children's hair?

Original horse shampoos may be too strong for children's hair. However, new formulations have been developed for all hair types. Equenne Mane and Tail is one horse shampoo which may be used on children's hair.

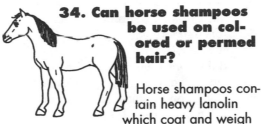

34. Can horse shampoos be used on colored or permed hair?

Horse shampoos contain heavy lanolin which coat and weigh the hair down, reducing the curl in your hair. This coating could also dull your color.

35. What makes the new horse shampoos different from shampoos made for humans?

They are generally thicker and more concentrated than human shampoo. Therefore, they are hard to rinse and can build up on the hair.

36. How should I correctly massage shampoo on my scalp?

Use your finger tips, never fingernails, to work shampoo on the scalp. You can also use a professional massage brush, such as J&D Massage Brush.

37. It never fails! By the end of the day I notice dandruff flakes in my hair. What type of shampoo will help?

Try a dandruff shampoo like Medi Dan, Medi Dan Extra or Queen Helene Dandruff Shampoo. They have an added ingredient that acts as a mild abrasive to shake dandruff loose from the scalp and wash it away. They are designed to remove OILY DANDRUFF not dry dandruff, which is typically caused by overuse of chemicals or styling aids. If dandruff is from dry scalp, you can use a dry scalp shampoo or moisturizing shampoo. Medi-Dan Dry Scalp Shampoo and other moisturizing shampoos, such as Ion Moisturizing Shampoo and Keragenics Therapy, will add moisture to scalp and hair. No dandruff shampoo will cure a medical skin condition, such as eczema or psoriasis. If you suspect this is the cause, consult your doctor or a dermatologist.

38. Can a dandruff shampoo be used every day?

Medi-Dan can be used every day, however there are five different formulas based on hair type. Be sure to select the formula best for you.

39. How often should I shampoo my hair if I have dandruff?

It depends on what type of dandruff you have. Medi-Dan Plus can be used every day because it has a conditioning formula. Stronger treatments, like Medi-Dan Extra, should not be used every day because it can be drying. This shampoo is best for dandruff combined with oiliness and flaking.

40. I have oily hair, but my scalp is dry and flaky. What shampoo should I use?

Medi-Dan Dry Scalp Shampoo will help alleviate the problem by cleansing hair well while still treating the scalp with medication to remove flakiness. Also try Fantasia IC 100% Pure Tea Shampoo.

41. How does salt water damage my hair, and what should I do to get it out of my hair?

When salt water dries on the hair it creates a high-saline solution which can cause mineral deposits to build up, resulting in hair that is weighted down and cannot grow. Hair should be washed or rinsed as soon as you get out of the water. Salon Care Ultra Moisturizing Anti-Chlorine Shampoo can remove salt water from hair.

42. My child's hair turned green from swimming all summer in the pool. What shampoo product can I use that will get rid of the green, yet not hurt my child's hair?

Salon Care Ultra Moisturizing Anti-Chlorine Shampoo or Action Environmental Pool & Spa Formula is gentle. It will remove the green after using one to six times, depending on the build-up.

43. I have permed and colored hair and will be swimming in the ocean on my vacation. What shampoo should I use that will wash out the salt, yet not strip my color?

Consider Action Environmental Pool & Spa Shampoo or Salon Care Anti-Chlorine Swimmers Shampoo. Both will remove salt without damaging color-treated hair.

F.Y.👁 What Is Hair?

Hair is made of a strong protein called "keratin," which contains 21 different amino acids. The hair shaft consists of the cuticle, the cortex and the medulla. The cuticle is the outer layer of the hair shaft, made of multiple layers of translucent cells which overlap each other like shingles on a roof. When the layers are smooth and flat against each other, the hair reflects more light and looks shiny. The middle layer of an individual hair is called the cortex which comprises three-quarters of the hair shaft. The pigment, or melanin, gives hair its color and is located in the cortex. There are two types of melanin: eumelanin, black pigment, and pheomelanin, red/yellow pigment. The core of the hair shaft is called the medulla.

44. If my hair has a squeaky feeling when I shampoo my hair, does this mean it is clean?

Squeaky clean indicates that oils have been removed from the hair. However, it also may indicate a raised hair cuticle. Rely on a thorough rinsing rather than that squeaky clean feeling.

45. What temperature should the water be when I rinse my hair after shampooing?

A cool water rinse helps close the cuticle, which makes the hair feel smoother. Hot water stimulates oil production, so if your hair is dry, you may want to use warm water. If hair tends to get oily quickly, cool or tepid water is recommended. The temperature should be determined by what you want to achieve.

46. Will rinsing your hair with cold water or vinegar after shampooing make your hair shiny?

Cool water and an acid vinegar rinse help to close the hair cuticle, making the hair appear shiny. Prepared finishing rinses are much easier to use, and they smell better, too! Try Ion Finishing Rinse.

47. How long should I rinse my hair after I shampoo?

The average time is 60-90 seconds. You know it is clean by the feel of your hair. Hair should not feel like it is coated. It is best to rinse hair with the water flowing in the direction of your cuticle, not against it—head is held back and water flows from forehead to back.

48. How should I treat my hair after I shampoo it?

Blot, don't rub hair dry, as rubbing can cause tangling. Comb hair with a wide-tooth comb, holding sections of hair to gently comb through tangles.

CHAPTER TWO

Treat Those Tresses

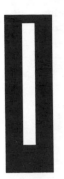

Imagine spreading a thick, greasy, gummy substance over your hair to condition it! That's what the ancient Egyptians did when they wanted to make their hair more manageable.

It was not uncommon to mix local fats and oils to create conditioners for the hair. One Egyptian solution consisted of a "mixture of six kinds of fat—the fat of a hippopotamus, a lion, a cat, a crocodile, a snake and an ibex."

Polynesians concocted a scented oil called "mouoi" and a gummy substance from the coconut tree called "pia" to create conditioners for the hair. The main problem with these early conditioners was they left the hair greasy, sticky and easily soiled.

It wasn't until the early 1950s when chemical suppliers realized that the technology used in fabric softeners to soften natural wool fibers could also be used in creating conditioners for the hair. These early conditioners were emulsions that contained oils, such as mineral oils. They looked similar to cream hairdressings, but they could be rinsed out without removing the good properties of the conditioners.

From magical mixtures of wild animal fats, hair conditioners have progressed beyond the greasy concoctions of Cleopatra's day. Today, there are thousands of conditioners on the market, all claiming to solve specific hair problems, if not ALL of them.

We expect a lot from conditioners. They should add moisture, strengthen hair, make it shinier, detangle it, smooth split ends, add fullness and body, and more.

Conditioners work in a variety of ways, some only working on the cuticle and others actually penetrating into the cortex for longer lasting results. These latter conditioners are called deep-penetrating "treatments" because they are used occasionally for therapeutic reasons.

Conditioning and shampooing go together like salt and pepper. However, shampoos don't take the place of conditioning. Shampoos clean. Conditioners NOURISH.

F.Y.👁 What Is A Humectant?

A humectant is an ingredient in hair products that draws moisture into the hair from the air. For dry hair, you want to be able to hold moisture. For fine, limp hair, you want to repel moisture. Humectants are also found in skin care products.

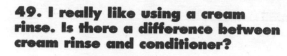

49. I really like using a cream rinse. Is there a difference between cream rinse and conditioner?

A cream rinse detangles and doesn't penetrate like a conditioner will. It works instantly, but must be rinsed out well or it leaves a residue, making hair look dull. A conditioner imparts moisture or protein to strengthen hair. Deep-penetrating conditioners actually penetrate the cortex.

50. What are some of the ingredients that make one conditioner different from another?

The formulation of moisturizers, proteins, botanicals and silicones vary among conditioners.

51. Why do so many conditioners and styling aids contain alcohol? Doesn't it dry hair out?

The kind of alcohol found in some shampoos and conditioners is cetyl or stearyl alcohol. This type actually helps condition hair to make it softer. Isopropyl alcohol is in hairspray and some other styling aids, and it is usually called "SD-40" alcohol on the label. It is the ingredient that makes hairspray dry quickly. Generally, there is not enough SD-40 alcohol in any professional beauty product to be harmful. But remember, over time, styling aids can build up and sap hair's moisture. Shampoo well and rinse thoroughly.

52. My hair is really damaged. Will it help to leave in a conditioner longer than the directions indicate?

Conditioners take a certain amount of time to penetrate the hair. After that time, there is no added benefit. Leaving a conditioner like a protein treatment in longer can actually do more harm than good by drying the hair out even more! Follow directions on the package or your stylist's advice.

53. I have an oily scalp, but my hair is dry. What conditioner will treat these opposing conditions?

Use a gentle cleansing shampoo, then apply a rinse-out conditioner, like Ion Moisturizing Treatment or Professional Prescription Enforce, working the conditioner well into the ends. Rinse thoroughly.

54. Why do some conditioners make your hair feel greasy?

The weight of the conditioner and its capacity to rinse out without any residue, rather than the amount used, contribute to that greasy feeling. Choose a lightweight conditioner, like a leave-in one, if the "greasies" are a concern.

55. Is it important to use the same brand of shampoo and conditioner?

Yes. For best results, use the same brand shampoo and conditioner because they are designed as a system to work in harmony. However, it is not absolutely necessary.

56. I think I have over-conditioned my hair. Help!

If hair is over-moisturized it is very limp. Hair that is over-proteined is brittle and hard. If you have either problem as a result of over-conditioning, use a clarifying shampoo.

57. What is a good "everyday" conditioner to use with an "everyday" shampoo?

Depending on the amount of conditioner needed, try Ion Finishing Rinse to make hair more manageable. Enforce by Professional Prescription offers more conditioning and can be used every day. Unicure Hair and Skin Conditioner is a good "everyday" conditioner for simply detangling. For economy, try Salon Care All-Purpose Remoisturizer in the gallon size. Other great everyday conditioners are Fermodyl Moisture Recovery Detangler, Acclaim Plus Daily Rinse Out Conditioner or Aura Rosemary & Mint Finishing Rinse.

58. Which is best, a leave-in or rinse-out conditioner?

Rinse-out conditioners do more permanent conditioning by filling in the cuticle or snags in the hair and making it stronger. Leave-in conditioners are made to maintain the hair on a daily basis. They make combing easier, which reduces friction, prevents breakage and adds sheen to the hair before drying. Leave-in conditioners also protect from additional moisture loss. Another type of leave-in conditioner, a perm rejuvenator, adds elasticity to the hair to encourage the curl pattern and add bounce. Moisturizers in the formula give the hair a healthy look.

59. Can leave-in conditioners be used on all textures of hair?

Yes. On fine, thin hair, leave-in conditioners condition without weighing hair down. On coarse, thick hair, the conditioning agents soften and make the hair easier to manage. Try Keragenics Rejuvenating Treatment, Infusium 23, Fantasia IC Hair and Scalp Treatment or Sheenique Stayz-N Leave-on Treatment.

60. I have fine hair. Should I avoid conditioners that weigh my hair down?

Conditioners of the past often seemed to plaster fine hair down on the head. Today, there are many lighter formulas. It may seem contrary to common sense, but a leave-in daily conditioner may actually work better for you than a rinse-out conditioner because it is formulated to be "lighter" on hair. Avoid conditioners that have waxy ingredients in them. Try using Jheri Redding Biotin or Volumizer Hydrating Leave In or Conditioner.

61. Why should I use an instant conditioner after I shampoo?

An instant conditioner smoothes the cuticle, making hair easy to comb. A smooth cuticle makes hair shine and look vibrant. Salon Care All Purpose Remoisturizer and Unicure Hair and Skin Conditioner both rinse out.

Leave-in conditioners include Ion Anti Frizz Leave In and Aphogee Pro Vitamin Leave In Treatment.

62. Can leave-in conditioners be used everyday?

Leave-in conditioners are made for daily use. Try Jheri Redding Biotin, Biotera Leave In, Aura Elixer and Volumizer Leave In.

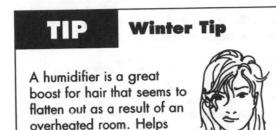

TIP   Winter Tip

A humidifier is a great boost for hair that seems to flatten out as a result of an overheated room. Helps beat flyaway hair, too!

63. I have oily hair. Should I use a conditioner?

Yes. It is best, however, to avoid using rinse-out conditioners. A leave-in conditioner or deep-penetrating treatment may be needed, especially if hair is permed or color-treated. Even oily hair can benefit from occasional moisturizing or protein treatments.

64. If I leave a conditioner on my hair longer than the instructions indicate on the package, will it condition my hair better?

No. The timing indicated on the package has been tested to determine when the product reaches its maximum effectiveness. For best results, follow directions closely.

65. If I use a moisturizing shampoo, should I use a conditioner?

Yes. There is little benefit to following a moisturizing shampoo with a rinse-out conditioner — that's two doses of the same medicine! A leave-in conditioner, however, can complement a moisturizing shampoo, and there are many products, like Volumizer Hydrating Leave-in Conditioner, designed to be used this way.

66. What is the best conditioner to use with a dandruff shampoo?

Generally a moisturizing treatment is best after using a dandruff shampoo. Try a leave-in treatment like Fantasia I.C. Hair & Scalp Treatment or Biotera Leave-in Conditioner.

67. What should I put on my hair before I wet comb it after shampooing so I will not break off my hair?

Use leave-in treatments, such as Jheri Redding Volumizer Leave In, Infusium 23, Ion Anti Frizz Leave In, Mixx Tangle Tonic, or Biotin Leave In Treatment, for hair that needs extra nourishing and is thin, fine or weak.

68. I have static in my hair. What can I do?

Look for a product that will give a slight coating to the hair. Try a spray-on, leave-in conditioner. Most conditioners will help reduce static. Good products to try include Influx CHP Vitamin Treatment, Keragenics Rejuvenating Treatment, Aura Elixer or Ion Anti Frizz Leave In Conditioner.

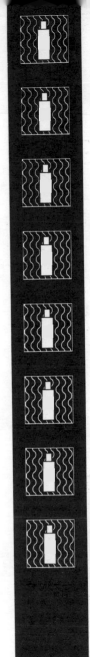

69. My hair goes limp in the mountains. What conditioner or treatment can I use that will bring it back to life?

Use a rinse-out moisturizing treatment, such as Ion Moisturizing Treatment, once a week, and a daily leave-in treatment to lock in moisture.

70. My hair tangles easily. What will take out the tangles, but not weigh down my thin hair.

Leave-in conditioners, like Jheri Redding Volumizer, Ion Anti Frizz Leave In Conditioner, and Infusium 23, are light formulas that will not weigh hair down. Also consider using Keragenics Revitalizing Protein Pac because it has panthenol to help re-moisturize hair.

71. I want to control my frizzy, fly-away hair. What can I use?

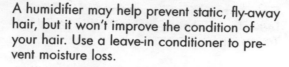

Frizzy hair is often caused by dryness. Use a light moisturizer after every shampoo. Try Ion Anti Frizz Leave In, Keragenics Rejuvenating Treatment or Apple Pectin Scentsates Conditioner.

72. I live in an extremely dry climate. Will a humidifier improve the condition of my hair?

A humidifier may help prevent static, fly-away hair, but it won't improve the condition of your hair. Use a leave-in conditioner to prevent moisture loss.

73. Is it okay to use conditioner every day on naturally curly hair?

Yes. Generally this type of hair requires more moisture.

74. Is a protein treatment the same as a conditioner?

Yes. Some conditioners work only on the hair's cuticle. These can be used every day. Protein treatments rebuild strength in hair that has lost its elasticity by adding protein to the cortex, allowing hair to be strong and retain moisture. These deep-penetrating treatments often come in single applications, in packets or vials. These treatments are designed for periodic use.

75. Will certain treatment products make my hair grow faster?

No. There is no over-the-counter treatment that can make hair grow faster.

76. Can a protein treatment be used on all textures of hair?

Yes. However, to be most effective, protein treatments should be used on damaged hair. Healthy, coarse hair is already strong and may only need extra moisture.

77. How many times should you use a protein treatment?

It depends on the hair damage. If a protein treatment is used too often, the hair can become dried out. As a general rule, it is safe to use a treatment weekly for the first month to get hair in good shape. Then, use it one or two times a month after that. Always follow the directions on the package or consult your stylist.

78. A stylist told me that constantly pulling back my hair in a ponytail or using hot rollers too much can put me at risk for hair loss. What should I use to build strength and resilience?

First, be sure you are using protected hair bands to help minimize hair breakage. Strengthen hair by periodically using protein treatments, such as Jheri Redding Natural Protein, Aphogee Protein Packs, Pantresse Vitamin Treatment Pack or Keragenics Revitalizing Protein Packs. All add tensile strength to keep hair from breaking.

79. The last time I got a perm, my hair was extremely brittle afterwards. What can I use before I get my next perm to avoid this problem?

Use a protein treatment at least three times a week and a moisturizing conditioner after you shampoo on the other days prior to perming. A daily moisturizing treatment such as Quantum Daily Moisturizing Treatment or Ion Moisturizing Treatment should help. For protein, try Ion Reconstructor, Fantasia IC Reconstructor or Jheri Redding Professional Prescription Curative Strengthening Treatment.

80. How often should I use a deep-penetrating protein treatment?

This type of treatment may be used once or twice a week, depending on the damage to your hair. Try it once a week for a month until hair is healthy. Then use the treatment once or twice a month thereafter. Overuse can be harmful to hair and dry it out.

81. My conditioner has placenta in it. What is the ingredient, and why is it important for hair?

This ingredient is known as "placentaisan amino acid" which is a protein complex to replenish moisture and protein in the hair. Try Fermodyl 07 or Beyond Belief #777 Ampoules.

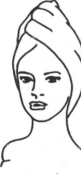

82. When using a deep-penetrating conditioner, why should I cover or wrap my head?

Keeping the head warm helps open the cuticle layer and allows the conditioner to penetrate more effectively. Your head can be wrapped with a hot towel or even plastic wrap. For easy, no-mess cover-ups, try plastic processing caps like your stylist uses, available at your local beauty supply store.

83. I never have time to deep-condition my hair. When is best, morning or night?

It doesn't matter. You can and should condition anytime. If you want to save time, you may want to condition while showering, wearing a plastic cap on the head so the conditioner penetrates better. A daily leave-in conditioner is a great answer to protecting hair from daily abuse of sun, wind and hot styling appliances.

84. I like to take steam baths and saunas. Will this help or harm my hair? What product could I use while doing this?

A sauna or steam bath will not harm your hair. Take advantage of the opportunity to condition your hair with a protein conditioner. After shampooing hair, apply conditioner and let it penetrate the hair as you enjoy your sauna or steam.

85. Should you shampoo after deep-conditioning to remove residue?

No. Shampooing after deep-conditioning counteracts the conditioning process. All shampoos contain lauryl sulfate, which removes oil from the hair.

86. I am going skiing this winter. When should I have a deep-conditioning treatment?

Conditioning should be planned monthly to

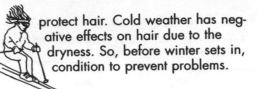

protect hair. Cold weather has negative effects on hair due to the dryness. So, before winter sets in, condition to prevent problems.

87. When I am under a lot of stress, my hair looks stressed out too! What type of treatment will revitalize my hair?

If hair is stressed because of overprocessing, you need a deep-penetrating treatment. If hair is simply dry, a deep-moisturizing treatment should be used, such as Ion Moisturizing Treatment, Salon Care Cholesterol Treatment or Quantum Extra Care Weekly Hair Repair. For every day, try Keragenics Rejuvenating Treatment because it contains panthenol and is effective on all hair types.

88. My hair is damaged from overprocessing. What conditioner will put moisture and bounce back into it?

Most hair damaged by overprocessing needs a combination of moisture and protein. The protein packs are excellent. Use a deep-penetrating conditioning treatment, such as Keragenics Revitalizing Protein Pac, L'Oreal Ineral Hair Fixer, Ion Effective Care & Intensive Therapy Conditioner Protein Pack and Aphogee Reconstructor Pack. For dry hair, use a deep-penetrating moisturizing treatment. For hair breakage, try a deep-penetrating protein treatment. If it is dry and brittle, it probably needs a strong moisturizing treatment left on for at least 15 minutes. On a day-to-day basis, a leave-in

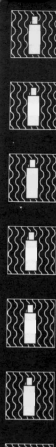

conditioner protects hair by sealing the cuticle to keep hair from being damaged further as it is brushed, combed or styled.

89. How does chlorine affect the condition of the hair?

Chlorine causes oxidation and oxidation by-products which cause dryness and lightening of the hair. To prevent this, use an anti-chlorine product, like Salon Care Ultra Moisturizing Shampoo and Conditioner after exposure to chlorine.

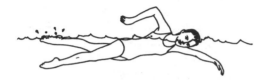

90. When is the best time to apply a conditioner to the hair after hair has been colored?

It is best to apply conditioner immediately after coloring. Use a deep-conditioner, like Wella pH-D In Depth Conditioner, Roux Mendex, Acclaim Plus KBF Reconstructing Treatment or Fermodyl Treatment Vial Special Formula, which is formulated for use on color-treated hair.

91. My scalp itches in the winter. What conditioner can I use to relieve the itching?

Try a hot oil treatment like Keragenics Hot Oil, which will moisturize the scalp and remove that itchy feeling. Aura Rosemary & Mint Rinse contains peppermint which soothes and cools itchy scalp.

92. Can a person with thin, fly-away hair use a hot oil treatment?

Yes. The results, however, will be minimal because hot oil treatments are topical and can weigh hair down. Fine hair needs a protein treatment to build strength, like Keragenics Liposome Hot Oil Treatment and Aphogee Evening Primrose Hot Oil Treatment, which rinse clean.

93. I have a hard time managing my shoulder-length curly hair. Any advice?

Use a leave-in conditioner to maintain moisture and control, like Revlon's Moisture Recovery 2-Phase Treatment or Ion's Anti-Frizz Leave-In Conditioner.

94. My hair is very thick. What conditioning product will actually make it behave as if it were thinner?

Check out a leave-in conditioner, like Keragenics Rejuvenating Treatment, to make hair more manageable.

95. Does a no-heat activated conditioner work as well as a heat-activated conditioner?

It depends on what you are trying to achieve. For damaged hair, a heat-activated conditioner may be more effective because heat tends to swell the cuticle allowing the conditioner to penetrate the hair more readily. Ion Microwave Treatment, Ion Hot Oil, Let's Jam

Hot Creme Treatment, L'Oreal Oleocap Lusterizer, Salon Care Cholesterol and Tresemme 4+4 Hot Oil are excellent options.

96. What is a scalp "facial"?

It is a detoxifying salon treatment that consists of massage, perhaps steam, and applying special cleansers, essential oils and moisturizers.

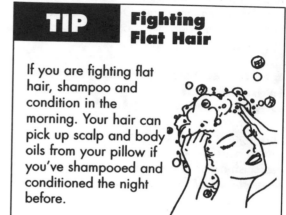

TIP | **Fighting Flat Hair**

If you are fighting flat hair, shampoo and condition in the morning. Your hair can pick up scalp and body oils from your pillow if you've shampooed and conditioned the night before.

97. What is the difference between a conditioner and a reconstructor?

A conditioner is often designed to add shine and manageability. The term "reconstructor" is used when the product has a high protein content to help strengthen hair. Examples of reconstructors are Aphogee Conditioning Treatment, Acclaim Plus KBF Reconstructor, L'Oreal Ineral Hair Fixer and Jheri Redding Keratin Reconstructor.

98. When should I use a reconstructor?

A reconstructor is best used weekly to repair protein damage caused by chemical services or heat styling. Use once a month to maintain healthy hair. Try Ion Reconstructor or Aphogee Conditioning Treatment.

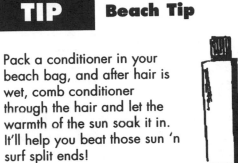

TIP   **Beach Tip**

Pack a conditioner in your beach bag, and after hair is wet, comb conditioner through the hair and let the warmth of the sun soak it in. It'll help you beat those sun 'n surf split ends!

99. My hair is thin and fine. Do I need a hair texturizer or hair thickener?

Both would work well, but differently. A texturizer styling lotion, such as Natural Balance Texturizing Setting Lotion, adds body and fullness and works well on most hair types. A thickener adds diameter to the hair by swelling the hair shaft. A good one to try is Fantasia Thick N' Hair or Acclaim Plus Body Builder, which adds fullness and body while conditioning.

100. Because my hair is so thin, I continually have split ends. Is there something I can put on my hair to keep the ends from appearing split?

Condition and trim hair on a regular basis. Minimize the use of excess heat on hair with blow dryers, hot rollers and curling irons. Use a thermal styling lotion, like Keragenics Heat Guard or Revlon Fermodyl Moisture Recovery 2-Phase Treatment, before blow drying or using hot rollers. For instant results, try a hair shiner, which is a silicone-based product used by rubbing onto ends of hair and styling. Shiners not only close the cuticle, but also fill in gaps where it is broken. They won't solve the problem, but they make hair look shinier and softer. Try Ion Anti Frizz Hair Glosser, Replenishing Hair Shiner by Jheri Redding Professional Prescription or Jheri Redding Volumizer Spray-on Shine. Be sure to follow directions. A tiny bit is all you need!

101. If I rub a fabric softener on my hair, will it condition my hair and eliminate static?

The fabric softener may eliminate hair static, but it provides no conditioning benefits to hair. In fact, it may leave a waxy coating that dulls the hair. Try Moisture Recovery Detangler, which leaves hair soft, manageable AND static-free.

102. When should I use a hair rinse or lemon rinse instead of conditioner? Will a vinegar rinse work as well?

Hair texture is the key. On fine hair, a lemon or vinegar rinse leaves hair with less tangles, but it could be too acidic for some fragile hair. Professional finishing rinses like Ion Finishing Rinse or Aura Rosemary & Mint Rinse offer the proper acid balance without the softening effect of a conditioner. Conditioners work best on hair that needs softening and manageability.

103. Is there such a thing as a "mask" for your hair?

Yes. Mud packs, however, provide only temporary topical help. Try Naturonics Organic Mud Treatment, available in individual packs and 12 ounce size. It is formulated with vitamins, minerals and botanical extracts to help restore moisture content and improve elasticity.

104. How can I make my naturally curly hair shine?

Try a silicone-based shiner, like Volumizer Spray-On Shine.

105. Should raw eggs be used to condition and style hair?

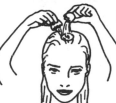

No. The protein molecules in eggs are too large to be absorbed by the hair.

106. I have hard tap water which dulls my hair. What can I do to improve the luster of my hair?

Minerals in hard water, like calcium and iron, bond to hair's protein making it dry and dull. Try Quantum Clarifying Shampoo or Action Environmental Hard Water Shampoo to remove hard water build-up.

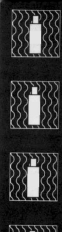

107. What are the benefits of using oils like olive oil or mayonnaise to condition my hair?

These oils moisturize and increase shine, making brittle hair more manageable, but are too heavy for most hair types, difficult to rinse out, and leave a heavy residue. For best results, however, use professional formula conditioners.

108. What medications affect the condition of my hair?

Most all do. Medications are excreted through the hair, leaving a fine, thin film on hair. Consider trying a clarifying shampoo to remove chemical traces from hair, especially before a perm or chemical services to improve results.

109. What can I do to repair fine, thin hair after my hair thinned out from a sickness and did not grow back to its original fullness?

First, consult your doctor. You might also try a regime formulated for thin hair like VazoCure System Kit. VazoCure BioStyme Scalp Treatment contains vasodilators that promote healthy hair growth by stimulating blood circulation. VazoCure ProFoam Protein Conditioning Treatment is a blend of proteins that help strengthen and increase hair's diameter.

110. Does soft water affect the condition of my hair?

The salt used in water softeners can cause build-up over time. Remove with a clarifying shampoo periodically.

F.Y. 👁 The Lowdown On Conditioners

Conditioners are designed to do a variety of things for your hair. Some work only on the cuticle and can be used every day. Other deep-penetrating treatments actually penetrate the cortex for longer lasting results and should be used only occasionally for extremely damaged hair.

Deep-penetrating treatments are often packaged as single-application packets or vials, because a little goes a long way! All actually open the cuticle to let moisture or protein into the cortex, the middle part of hair that gives it strength and retains moisture. Some treatments require heat, i.e., sitting under a dryer, wearing a heat cap or wrapping the head. These are the most powerful conditioners.

There are two basic types of deep-penetrating treatments: moisturizing and protein. Moisturizing treatments put moisture, softness and "bounce" back into hair that's dried out from overprocessing, heat styling or exposure to sun and wind. HOT OIL and CHOLESTEROL products are two types of moisturizing treatments, though there are others.

Protein treatments may also be called "protein packs." They rebuild strength in hair that has lost its elasticity by adding protein to the cortex. Often this treatment is given before a perm or hair color service to get hair in the best shape. Protein treatments are excellent when used as needed, but overuse without the proper moisture balance can severely dry hair.

Moisturizing and protecting are also attainable with daily conditioners, but they are not as strong as the deep-penetrating treatments. They are commonly called rinse-out or leave-in conditioners.

CHAPTER THREE

Spritz, Sprays, Shiners 'n Gels

Today's styling products are a far cry from 1500 B.C. when the Assyrians first began styling hair as a profession. In fact, the Assyrians developed hair styling to the exclusion of nearly every other cosmetic art!

Not surprisingly, the Greeks of the Homeric Period believed that elaborate and complex hairstyles denoted culture and distinguished them from the northern barbarians.

Fair hair was preferred, and perhaps one of the earliest styling products was a talc consisting of yellow flour and fine gold dust which was used to lighten the hair. Dusting hair in various colored powders was the height of fashion in 16th century France. By the 1790s, the court of Marie Antoinette made powdering and all types of hairdressings the rage. Hair was combed, curled, waved, and piled high with false hair into towers that were then powdered in a myriad of colors.

Powder has gone the way of the guillotine, only to be replaced by the most high-tech of styling products that can shape, mold, wave, scrunch, curl and hold hair through the strongest of gale force winds.

There are gels, glazes, mousses, spritzes, sprays, shiners, stylers and waxes to create any look imaginable. And credit goes to the hairdresser, in most cases, who often conceived these products with an eye to the creativity and flexibility they would provide.

111. What is the difference between mousse, liquid, lotion, spritz, spray gel, glaze and gel?

Mousse is a light hold, fast drying foam. Use on wet or dry hair. Mousse adds lift and fullness and can protect against heat and dryness. Styling liquids, lotions and creams are medium-hold products worked through wet hair with the hands. They add volume, shape or style, control curls and define spiked styles. Spritzing the base of hair helps it stand up from the roots and appear fuller. Spritz and spray gels are pump sprays usually used on dry or damp hair to sculpt or control it. They add body and texture. Spritzes tend to be stiffer than spray gels. Spray gels can achieve the wet look. Glazes and gels are thick liquids used on wet or dry hair. Use for sculpting wet looks, for accenting particular curls or controlling thick, wavy hair.

TIP Tips On Twists

Those sophisticated updos are ever-so-easy when you use gels, styling sprays and mousse to add structure and hold. Mousse makes hair easier to shape into chignons or French twists and provide excellent hold.

112. I have very fine, thin hair, but my hair needs a lift! What type of styling product should I use?

Mousses work best for adding fullness and giving hair a lift. By applying it to the scalp, it can produce more fullness when damp hair is blown dry. Try using Jheri Redding Volumizer Mousse, Volumax Mousse, Ion Alcohol Free Mousse or Aura Lemon Grass Mousse. A firm hold hairspray will help keep fine hair in place.

113. I have limp hair and maxed out highlights, what can I do to give my hair a lift?

Try a color-enhancing mousse, like Roux Fancifull Mousse, which adds highlights as well as body and volume.

114. Is it better to use mousse or gel to style your hair, and when do you apply them, before or after blow drying?

A mousse or gel should be applied to the hair before blow drying. Most have an ingredient that helps to protect the hair from the heat of the blow dryer. When applying a mousse or gel after blow drying, re-wet the hair to build extra body. Be aware, however, that you may not end up with the desired result because the hair may get weighed down or flattened if you apply these styling aids after blow drying. Good products to try are Jheri Redding Volumizer Mousse to add body, Ion Mousse for fine hair, Avec Mousse, Tresemme 4+4 Mousse and Net Effect Styling Mousse Stiff. Spray gels tend to work better on fine hair, because the spray allows for more even distribution. Try Volumizer Spray Gel. Thicker styling gels, like Jheri Redding Alcohol Free Styling Gel, Ion Anti Frizz Styling Gel and Salon Care Aloe Styling Gel are best used when firm control and hold or a wetter look are desired. They also add body to the ends of hair.

115. Gels thicken up and make my hair look dull. What can I use that will hold my hair, yet look soft?

Mousse is probably your best bet. It is the lightest hold, yet most versatile styling aid. Use on wet or dry hair, overall, to fluff up and add volume, or apply it to the sides of hair for a slicked-back look. You can also apply it just to the roots to make hair stand away from the head and appear fuller. Mousse is easy to use and combines some of the hold of a gel, with a softer, more natural feel. It can also work as a thermal protector to help shield hair from the heat of curling irons and blow dryers.

116. I would like to try a mousse to add body to my thin hair. How much should I use for short hair, medium-length hair or long hair?

For short hair, use a golf ball-size puff of mousse. For shoulder-length hair, fill the palm with mousse. For long hair, cover the palm and fingers with the mousse.

117. I want to add body to my hair, but don't want a perm. What should I do?

Try having hair cut in layers and using a mousse, gel or product designed specifically to add body to hair, like Acclaim Plus Body Builder.

118. I live in a hot, humid climate and have very frizzy hair. What products will help me manage the frizzies?

A silicone shiner in drop or spray formulation helps seal the cuticle to prevent moisture from entering the hair, which causes it to frizz. Try Ion Anti-Frizz Glosser or Hask Pure Shine Spray On.

119. Can you use a mousse on your hair if you have already used a conditioner?

Yes, you can use a mousse because it is a styling product. For light support, try Net Effect Mousse or Ion Alcohol-Free Styling Mousse. For more support, try Volumizer Mousse or Tresemme 4+4 Mousse.

120. Which styling product is least drying—a mousse or gel?

Gels tend to have more water, making them less drying. Consider using Ion Alcohol-Free Mousse or Jheri Redding Professional Prescription Alcohol-Free Styling Gel. Fantasia Liquid Mousse is also alcohol-free and contains panthenol for a healthy, shiny look.

121. How can I revive my style at the end of the day?

Brush through dry hair or retouch it with a damp comb, then spray again with hairspray. If you already have gel in your hair and want to revive your style, try spraying on a leave-in conditioner to reactivate the gel, then restyle hair. Leave-in treatments include Ion Anti Frizz, Keragenics Leave In or Biotera Leave In.

122. What is the best way to apply gel to hair?

Apply gel first to the hands, rubbing gel on palms and fingers, then apply to the roots of the hair from the underside. If you apply gel through to the ends, you can weigh the hair down.

TIP   Frizz Fighter

Shine products in easy spray-on applicators make fighting the frizzies a breeze. The secret's in the silicone which causes the hair cuticle to lie flat. When using a rub-on shine product, use only a tiny amount on the palm. Rub into hands and on finger tips, then rub over surface of the hair or on frizzy ends. Voila!

---

123. What is the best product to use for naturally curly hair after shampooing? Gel, mousse or spray?

All three products can be used, depending on the look you want to achieve. Consider this when making your choice: gels, when applied to the root area, give maximum control and lift at the scalp, allowing for free-falling curls with volume. Apply gel throughout hair for a sleeker, straighter style. Try Professional Prescription or Tresemme 4+4 Styling Gel.

124. What is the proper amount of gel to use on hair?

Use about a quarter-size amount of gel on short or medium-length hair. Double that amount for long hair, but apply only about half that amount to the hair first, then apply the rest so that the product is evenly distributed throughout the hair.

125. I have a problem restyling my hair after I've gelled it. My hair is so stiff, it pulls when I brush it. What should I do to avoid hair breakage?

You may be using too much gel or a product that is too strong. The problem could also be that the product is not evenly distributed throughout hair. Try using a glaze, like Tresemme 4+4 Glaze, instead of a gel. You could also try using a leave-in conditioner before adding gel to the hair to provide more manageability, making it easier to comb hair after it dries.

126. I love the natural look. How do I finger sculpt or scrunch curls in my hair? What product is best to use?

Generally, a gel, spray gel or mist-type gel product works best for finger sculpting. To achieve this look, simply spray gel all over head, or work a regular gel evenly throughout hair. Lift curls at the base and continue lifting as the hair dries. Lifting is important because the moisture in the hair can weigh it down. What you are trying to do is lift the curl formation closer to the roots which achieves that "scrunched" look. Try Ion Anti Frizz Gel or Jheri Redding Spray Gel in the Volumizer line.

127. My hair has a slight curl, making it hard for me to style. What product can help me manage my hair better?

First apply a leave-in conditioner to damp hair. Then apply a spray-on gel, like Revlon Moisture Recovery or Volumax Spray Gel, and scrunch hair into place.

128. I like the look of the flip, what can I use?

Use a glaze on the ends of the hair for maximum hold. Work a small amount through the last 2 to 3 inches of hair length and shape hair into a flip. Try Biotera Styling Glaze.

129. What product can I use when I blow dry my hair near my part to add more volume at the crown?

Blow dry hair until it is completely dry. Then re-spray the part area with a root-lifting product, such as a spray gel, and lift hair with fingers. Let hair air dry. Try Jheri Redding Volumizer Spray Gel or For Perms Only Spray Gel.

130. How do I get a really wavy look without a perm?

A wavy look requires a curl formation where the base of the curl is directed in alternating directions. For example, one row of curls is directed to the right, the next row to the left. Styling gels hold waves that are combed into short hair. Wave clamps work well to hold the waves in place until hair dries.

131. What styling aid do I use to achieve the wet look?

Spray gels, glaze or gels achieve this wet look. Try Tresemme 4+4 Glaze, Professional Prescription Gel, Queen Helene Styling Gel, Biotera Gel or Volumax Glaze. Apply to damp hair and allow to dry. Do not comb or brush after drying.

132. I love the extra hold that gels offer, but hate the stiff, dull finish. What should I use that is light, yet leaves shine in my hair?

Use gels that are clear to give hair better shine. Use less of a gel product, or add water to the gel to reduce the stiffness. Good ones to try are Professional Prescription Styling Gel and Hair Fixative by Jheri Redding, Salon Care Aloe Vera Styling Gel and Tresemme 4+4 Styling Gel.

TIP **Stand Out Tips**

Create the illusion of thicker hair by making hair stand out, not lie flat. Brush **chin-length** hair away from face with a flat brush, then apply mousse sparingly to hair. Bend over and blow dry hair flat and up, beginning at the nape of the neck. Smooth into style.

---

133. What is a styling glaze, and how should it be used?

Styling glaze is a firm-hold styling product that should be distributed evenly through wet hair. Use instead of a styling gel or other set

ting product. Try Volumax Glaze, Tresemme 4+4 Styling Glaze or Biotera Styling Glaze.

134. My hair is so thick that it will not hold a curl. What styling product can I use that will help my hair hold curl?

For wet styling, use a strong-hold styling lotion, like Tresemme 4+4 Glaze and a roller set. For dry styling, spray hair with a firm styling spray, like Volumizer Working Spray, Tresemme 4+4 Brush Out Working Spray, or Acclaim Plus KBF Spray before using curling appliances. This will create longer lasting curls.

135. I have flyaway hair, but love the look of "finger" or "molded" waves. Is there any hope for me?

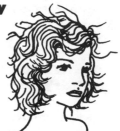

Yes! Styling aids such as gels and glazes will help control flyaway hair. Try Ion Design Sculpting Lotion or Tresemme 4+4 Styling Glaze for finger or molded waves. Also, hair shiners can keep those stray hairs under control. Anti Frizz Gloss will help keep flyaway hair from becoming such a headache.

136. What is a thermal styling lotion, and when should it be used?

Thermal lotions are specifically formulated to protect hair from blow dryer, curling iron and hot roller damage. Use a product like Keragenics Heat Guard or Fantasia Ultra

High Heat Styling Mist before blow drying or rolling with hot curlers. Leave-in conditioners like Fantasia IC Hair & Scalp Treatment or Sheenique Stayz-N Treatment also work well.

137. What styling product should I use with my hot rollers to protect my hair from heat damage?

Thermal styling lotions are designed to be used with styling appliances, like hot rollers. Consider also using a spray gel for a crisper set or a mousse for softer set. Styling products made especially for rollers and hot rollers include Fantasia Ultra High Heat Styling Mist and Isoplus Hot, Hot Curler.

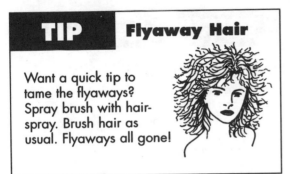

TIP Flyaway Hair

Want a quick tip to tame the flyaways? Spray brush with hairspray. Brush hair as usual. Flyaways all gone!

138. What are setting lotions, and how are they used?

Setting lotions are medium-hold products designed to be worked through wet hair with the hands. They add volume, shape and style, control curls or define "spiked" styles. Good ones to try are Resque Ultimate Styling and Sculpting Lotion and Natural Balance Setting and Texturizing Lotion, and Acclaim Plus Setting Lotion.

139. Is the silicone in my hair shiner harmful?

No. Most hair shiners contain water soluble silicone that improves the appearance of split ends and provides dramatic improvements fast. Silicone closes the hair cuticle and fills in gaps where it is broken. Try Volumizer Spray In Shiner, Frizz Care or Aphogee Gloss Therapy.

140. My hair looks dull. What can I do to create more shine?

Hair shiners that spray on, rub on or are worked through the hair contain silicone or cyclomethicone that add shine to hair. They can be used before or after hairspray, but preferably before. Good ones to try are Aphogee Gloss Therapy, ACV Gloze Therapy Gloss, Ion Anti Frizz Glosser and Professional Prescription Replenishing Hairshiner. Spray-on formulas include Hask Pure Shine, Volumizer Spray On Shine and Frizz Care. The key is to use shiners VERY SPARINGLY! A little dab does it!

141. Should a shiner be applied on wet or dry hair?

Hair can be dry or slightly damp. If you are doing a French braid, you want hair slightly damp. If hair will be in a style that moves, shiner should be applied on dry hair as a finishing product.

142. Should shiners be applied on the hair or at the roots?

Generally, they are used to add shine to the hair, and thus, should be applied on the hair strand itself.

143. I've been using a shiner, but it makes my fine, thin hair look greasy. How can I prevent that greasy look?

The amount of shiner you use varies with the amount of hair you have and its texture. For medium-length hair, use about the size of a dime, applied to the middle of the palm of your hand. Rub on hands, then apply by wiping hands on the hair. For fine, thin hair try a spray-on shiner like Volumizer Spray On Shiner, Hask Pure Shine, Frizz Care and Let's Jam Oil Free Shiner.

144. What can I use to control my hair when I French braid it?

Try silicone shiners such as Ion Anti Frizz Glosser, Professional Prescription Replenishing Hair Shiner or Frizz Care Hair Treatment to hold hair together and keep loose ends from flying. When hair is braided wet, apply a gel first, then a secondary application of a hair shiner. If hair is braided when dry, silicone shiners work well.

145. What type of shiner is best for short hair?

Use a shiner in spray form because it will provide more even distribution. For light hold with shine, try Volumizer Extra Shine Polishing Gel.

146. What type of shiner should be used on long hair?

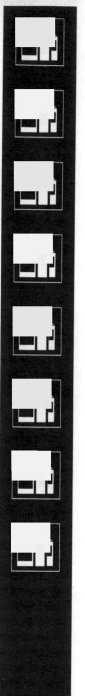

Liquid shiners work best on long hair because you can distribute them through the hair with your hands, paying particular attention to dry, troubled areas, such as the ends or at the hair line. Try Jheri Redding Replenishing Hair Shiner or ACV Gloze.

TIP   **Quick Pick Up**

Got a hot engagement after work and hair is limp and tired? Pep it up by first brushing through hair. Then section front and sides, tease slightly at roots and spritz or spray with a holding hairspray at the roots only. Smooth hair into style. Spray lightly again, if desired, to hold style.

147. I spritz my hair every morning, but it doesn't hold my set. What am I doing wrong?

It is easy to confuse spritz with hairspray, but there is an important difference. Spritz has holding resins like all styling support products. They add body and texture to a style. Hairsprays also have "memory" resins, which cause hair to "remember" the way it was styled and to return it to that style after it has been combed or fluffed. To hold your set, use a hairspray, like Grand Finale Hair Spray, Net Effect, Vita E or a Freezing Spray like Jheri Redding Volumizer.

148. Why does spritz make my hair look wet when I want a dry look?

A spritz or spray of any type should not make hair look wet unless it is being used too heavily or being sprayed too near hair. Spritz is a firm-hold and fast-drying spray that should be used SPARINGLY.

149. Is there a hairspray that can be used every day and won't coat your hair?

Some hairsprays are clean and tend to be less coating than others. A good example of this type of spray is Shaper Spray by Generics Value Products, which contains a clear base and does not dull the hair. Also try Ion Hair Spray in the non-aerosol formula. Avoid freezing sprays because they contain more resin and are more difficult to get out of the hair. Spritzing sprays are designed to coat the hair to add body.

150. Can styling gels be used over hairspray?

Yes, however, for best results you should use a spray gel first, then finish with a hairspray. The holding power of the gel will be increased by spraying over the gel.

151. What hairspray won't flake on my hair?

Clear-formula liquid sprays generally go on smoothly. Because they coat the hair only slightly, they tend to flake less. Flaking can also be caused by holding the spray too near the hair, resulting in a concentration of spray in one area. Ion Long-Lasting Liquid Hair Spray works well without flaking. If you prefer an aerosol, try Professional Prescription Ultra Control Hairspray or Vita E Hairspray. Both are clear aerosol formulas.

152. What is the best hairspray to use on gray hair to avoid yellowing?

Choose a clear formula with a UV protectant to prevent yellowing. Good ones to try are Quantum Finishing Spray, Acclaim Plus Hair Spray, or Tresemme 4+4 Fine Mist Spray.

153. Is there a light hairspray that also offers super hold?

The amount of hold provided by a hairspray is determined by the amount of resin in the product. Try Sheer Mist or Ion Hard-to-Hold hairspray.

TIP   **Using Styling Products**

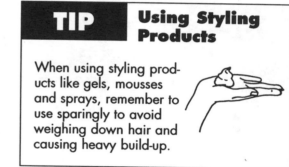

When using styling products like gels, mousses and sprays, remember to use sparingly to avoid weighing down hair and causing heavy build-up.

154. I live in California and have had trouble finding my favorite hairspray. Has it been discontinued?

California was one of the first states to limit levels of Volatile Organic Compounds (VOC's), like alcohols and certain types of propellants commonly found in hairsprays. Some manufacturers have chosen not to modify their products to comply with these California standards, and as a result, their products are not available there. Since the regulations, many new formulas have been developed by professional hair care companies. These products are available in many beauty supply stores.

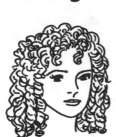
155. What is the difference between a "working" hairspray and a "freezing" hairspray?

A "working" spray contains flexible resins that do not dry as firmly as the freezing-type resins. Freezing sprays are very firm holding and are designed to keep hair in a "fixed" position.

156. What will keep my hair in one place ALL day?

Your best bet is a "freezing spray," which can also be used for spot styling or problem areas. Check out Avec Instant Ultimate Hold, Jheri Redding Volumizer Freeze Spray or Volumax Freezing Spray.

157. Will hairspray cause my hair to fall out?

There are no chemicals in hairsprays that will cause hair to fall out. If you used a "freezing spray" to hold hair in place all day, do not brush it out, just shampoo. Sometimes brush-ing through a "freezing spray" can put too much stress on your hair.

158. My hair is chemically processed. What type of hairsprays should I avoid?

Generally, avoid sprays with a high amount of resins or agents used for stiffening. These usually include freezing sprays. However, because most hairspray is water soluble, they can be washed out of the hair.

159. What hairspray can I use that will brush out easily?

Use a "working" type hairspray, such as Generics Shaper Spray, Biotera Shaping Spray or Tresemme 4+4 Brush Out Shaping Spray. Due to their quick-drying formulas and light hold, these sprays brush out easily. Also, AVEC Firm Hold and Aura Witch Hazel hair-spray brush out easily.

160. Which is better, a pump or aerosol spray?

Pump sprays go on wetter, and as a result, take longer to dry. Aerosols can provide more precise control for spot holding. It is really a matter of preference.

161. Is it damaging to comb or brush hair that has been sprayed with hairspray?

Yes. Combing or brushing hair after applying styling aids can break and split hair. Wet hair first, then comb or brush before styling. Let hair dry. Then reapply the styling product. Avoid overuse of styling products if you comb or brush your hair often during the day. Be sure to use a wide-tooth comb or pick, or brush with flexible ball-tipped bristles.

162. How can hat-flattened hair be spruced up?

Bend over and brush hair away from scalp. Spray root area with a spritz, like Tresemme 4+4. Gently lift hair and pick it into place with your fingers or feather comb it. Finish with a freezing spray such as Tresemme 4+4 or Jheri Redding Volumizer.

163. I hate build-up from styling products. Are there any that won't build up?

Most styling products are water soluble. With proper use and regular shampooing you can avoid build-up. It is a good idea to choose products from the same line because they are designed to work together, making it less likely they will build up.

 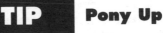
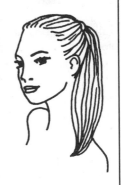

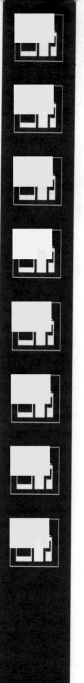

164. I noticed dandruff-like flakes after I started using a gel. Can I get dandruff from a styling product?

A styling product won't cause dandruff, but you can get flaking caused by an overuse of styling products. The best way to eliminate the problem is to use an everyday shampoo. Once a week or every two weeks, use a clarifying shampoo to get rid of styling product build-up.

165. What is the benefit of using styling products with sunscreen?

Styling products with sunscreens help protect hair from the sun's UV rays. As a result, they help keep hair from drying out or fading. Salon Care Quick Dry Sculpting Spray, and all Aura, Biotera and Acclaim Plus styling products contain sunscreens. For prolonged exposure to the sun, consider more protection, such as sprays, mousses, even conditioners. Reapply after swimming to maintain protection.

166. I have very thin hair. Should I consider semi-permanent custom hair extensions?

Hair extensions are artificial or human hairpieces that are braided, sewn, woven or glued onto hair. They last about six months and should be tightened every month. Although customized hair extensions can be costly and time-consuming, the look may be well worth the effort. Always consult a trained professional for this service. Temporary clip-in hair extensions are also available which blend into your natural hair color. Check your local beauty supply store.

167. What type of hair is used in hair extensions?

Most temporary hair extensions are made of 100% human hair from India or China. Because East Indian hair is finer than Chinese hair, it more closely resembles Caucasian hair. Many extensions are made of both East Indian and Chinese hair because the Chinese hair adds texture.

168. Can temporary hair extensions be permed and colored?

Yes. Consult a professional stylist for best results.

169. I like the look of sleek, slicked-back hair pulled into a tight chignon. What is the best product to use to create this look?

A glaze, like Tresemme 4+4, provides that clean, sleek look. You can also try a styling gel, like Jheri Redding Volumizer Polishing Gel to add extra shine.

170. What is spot styling?

Rather than using one product all over the hair, you use tiny amounts of several products on different sections of hair to achieve the desired result.

171. What is the benefit of silicone?

Silicone is an ingredient used in hair shiners to smooth the hair cuticle, making the hair easy to comb and leaving it silky and shiny.

172. How can I duplicate that bulky, textured look that my hairdresser gets after cutting my hair?

The new thickening hair creams add bulk and texture to any hair type. Unlike a styling product, they do not "hold" the hair in place, but rather make the hair feel "bulked up" and still moveable. Try Mixx Fanatical Hair Creme or Jheri Redding Volumizer Thickening Creme or Apple Pectin Scentsates Styling Cream.

Beauty Diary

SPRITZ, SPRAYS, SHINERS 'N GELS

Beauty Diary

SPRITZ, SPRAYS, SHINERS 'N GELS

CHAPTER FOUR

Tools Of The Trade

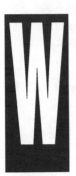

Where would the world be without a comb? Perhaps that question was asked more than 6,000 years ago when it is believed the first man-made combs were used by the ancient Egyptians. However, the most primitive comb dates back to 4,000 B.C. in Asia and Africa when a large, dried fish backbone served to groom and style hair.

Because the comb resembles teeth, it is not surprising that the word "comb" is derived from the ancient Indo-European term "gombhos," which means "teeth."

According to archeologists, with the exception of the Britons, all early cultures used combs. It was not until the Danes inhabited the British coastline in the mid-800s that the Britons were taught how to groom their hair regularly with a comb.

Like the comb, the hair pin has a history that goes back hundreds of years. This seemingly simple styling tool was used by the ancient Greeks and Romans, not to mention, Cleopatra, who preferred her hair pins in ivory and studded with jewels. In fact, the hair pin served a deathly dual purpose. Some were hollowed out to conceal poison, and it is believed that a hair pin of this design was used by Cleopatra when she poisoned herself.

Thankfully, today's modern hair styling tools are designed solely for the purposes of grooming and styling the hair. And they have expanded much beyond the earliest combs and hair pins to the most sophisticated of implements.

Professional styling tools range from a multitude of brushes, combs, clamps, rollers and ratts, picks and pins. Their usage is limited only by your imagination!

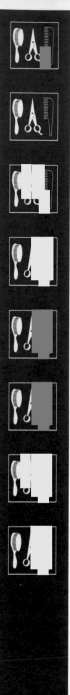

173. When should hair brushes be washed, and when should they be tossed?

Personal hair brushes should be washed on a routine basis, depending on the build-up of natural oils from the scalp and the use of styling products. Use a comb to remove hair from the bristles and wash the brush in warm water with mild soap or try Ship-Shape Brush and Comb Cleaner. Shake out excess water and air dry. Toss out when bristles begin to lose their stiffness or when a brush loses its effectiveness.

174. Why is there a hole in the cushion of my brush?

All professional-quality rubber cushion brushes are produced with a hole in the cushion so that air can circulate underneath and dry out the rubber. If there was not a hole, the cushion would trap the moisture, and eventually rot the rubber, ruining the brush.

175. What is meant by a professional brush?

Professional brushes are full-length brushes which usually feature six to seven rows of straight tufts of bristles. They are great for roller sets and general brushing, styling and finishing. Use on fine to medium hair textures. Try the Continental 5-Row Reinforced Boar Brushes or Lookin' Good 7-Row Reinforced Boar Brushes.

176. What are those round balls on the bristles of my hair brush?

The round balls are epoxy ball-tips. The brush is dipped into the epoxy which creates the tiny balls. They help the brush glide through the hair more easily and prevent abrasions to the scalp, breaking or pulling of the hair.

F.Y. 👁 Roller Rap

There are 10 basic types of rollers:
* Magnetic rollers are used for wet sets to add smooth curls and lots of body.
* Self-holding rollers, like Velcro-brand rollers, are used on damp or dry hair to create soft curls and full-bodied styles.
* Foam cushion rollers are best for fragile hair and for sleeping.
* Snap-on rollers are brush rollers encased in plastic that can be sterilized and used to securely hold hair.
* Snap-on magnetic rollers are made for fragile hair because they are gentle to hair and scalp.
* Plastic mesh rollers create smooth, beautiful curls and promote quick drying.
* Steam rollers steam in long-lasting curls.
* Wire mesh rollers, in which the metal wire heats up with the help of a dryer, create crisp curls.
* Brush rollers are designed to hold hair securely in place.
* Hair twirlers or flexi-rods create soft, natural curls without pins or clips and provide a variety of styles. They are specifically designed to create spiral curls.

---

177. If I own only one brush, what would be the best all-purpose brush to purchase?

A good cushion brush would be the best choice, such as the Spornette #25 combination boar and nylon pin bristle brush in a rubber cushion.

178. What is a boar bristle brush?

A boar bristle brush is one in which the filament or bristle comes from the wild boar. Usually the bristle comes from India or China where the animals are raised for their hair. Often, manufacturers reinforce the boar bristle with heat-resistant nylon to help the bristles penetrate the hair. Professional-quality brushes to try include Lookin' Good 7-Row 100% Boar Bristle Wave Brush and Phillips Super Round 100% Boar Bristle Brush. Reinforced boar brushes include Spornette RPB Round Brushes, Round Spornette RP10 Club and Continental's Reinforced Boar Brush.

179. Are natural bristle brushes better?

Natural bristles come from the wild boar and are softer and more flexible than nylon bristle and help to distribute the hair's natural oils throughout the hair. The bristles also help close the hair cuticle while brushing, giving the hair a nice, healthy shine. These types of brushes are more gentle on hair and scalp. Split ends and related hair damage are usually eliminated by using a boar bristle brush.

180. My stylist recommended I purchase a vent brush. What type of brush is this, and how should it be used?

A vent brush features openings in the back of the brush to allow air from the blow dryer to flow through. Drying and styling time is reduced using a vent brush, and it also creates volume for many hairstyles. Try the Original Bobby Vent Brush or the Phillips Hot Styler with aluminum insert on the base. This base absorbs heat from your blow dryer to speed up drying time.

181. What type of brush will make my hair shine?

Boar bristle brushes make hair shine because they help pick up and distribute the hair and scalp's natural oils along the hair shaft as well as pull dirt or dust particles off the hair. A good one to try is Spornette #25 Porcupine Boar Brush.

182. If I brush my hair every day for at least 15 minutes, will it make my hair grow?

Brushing stimulates circulation in the scalp, bringing more blood to the surface, which may stimulate hair growth. The more often you brush, the more oils you distribute from your scalp to the hair strands, which condition and protect the hair. As a result, hair is stronger and healthier.

183. When should I use a nylon bristle brush and when should I use a boar bristle brush?

A nylon bristle brush is best used on thick hair and to help detangle hair. Use a boar bristle brush for brushing out a style to create a fuller look. Boar bristle brushes are great to use at night to brush hair out for healthy shine.

184. I have flyaway hair. What is the best type of brush for eliminating static?

Try an anti-static or static-free brush. This type of brush has been made by blending carbon into the plastic. Brushes made entirely of wood generally are more static-free than others. Good static-free brushes to try include Cricket Fast Flow Ultra Vent, and RPM Round Brushes, Continental W-Back Vent and Tunnel Vent Brushes.

TIP | **Curl Hair Without Frizzing**

Coax curl into hair without frizzing it by drying hair with a diffuser. Bend over and keep head down while holding diffuser upward toward the scalp, trapping heat in the hair. With other hand, gently scrunch (or wrinkle) hair, pushing it up toward the scalp. Toss head back, and with dryer on coolest setting, use fingers to comb hair back away from face. Fluff out with pick if desired and spray with light-holding spray to finish style.

---

185. What type of hair is best suited to a full, round spiral brush?

It can be used on most textures and lengths of hair, but is best on short or layered hair. Because of the spiral, be careful not to completely rotate the brush in your hair or you will cause tangles. The diameter of the barrel determines the size of the resulting curl. Never pull the brush out of the hair. Try the Conair Elegante Spiral Brush.

186. What type of hair tool can be used to give me the same effect as a roller?

If you are looking for a non-electrical tool, try a barrel-shaped brush with a metal core designed to be used with a blow dryer. It is available in a variety of sizes to achieve many of the looks rollers provide and can be used on all hair lengths. Good ones to try are Spornette Magna Barrel, Modena or Taegu Round Brush.

187. I would like to set my hair with Velcro rollers, but don't have the time every day to let the hair air dry. What is the best option for me?

A round brush used with a blow dryer on cool setting would speed up drying time without damaging the hair.

188. What is the best brush for very thick, straight hair?

A rubber cushion brush with nylon bristles and ball-tip ends is your best bet. The rubber cushion helps make brushing easier, while the nylon bristles provide the strength to move the brush through thick hair. The ball-tips help reduce drag and resistance. Try the Jerome Alexander Jumbo Paddle Brush, the Phillips Avante Garde or Beautique Oval Cushion Brush.

189. I have curly hair. What is the best brush for me?

Generally, curly hair should not be brushed unless you intend to straighten it. In this case, the best brush is a natural reinforced boar bristle brush, such as Spornette RPB Round Brush or the Beautique Reinforced Boar Rounder.

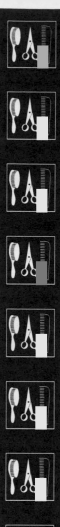

190. My hair is board straight. What is the best brush for me?

Use a brush that is gentle to the hair to prevent damage. Brushes with cushion bases and ball-tip bristles are best. Available in a variety of sizes and shapes for short to long hair, these brushes include the Slimline Cushion Brush assortment and the Curlmaster Paddle Brush. Ball-tipped vent brushes are recommended for blow dry styling.

191. What is the best brush for fine, thin hair?

Use a wide-spaced, ball-tipped bristle brush. This will prevent breakage and add lift and volume while blow drying. Try the Cricket Static-Free Brush, the Static-Free Fast-Flow Brush, the Beautique Tunnel Vent Brush or Continental Tunnel Vent Brush.

192. What brush is the best for a flip or pageboy?

Try a half-round twist brush if your hair is medium to thick. The twist design enables the bristles to provide total coverage when brushing the hair or styling in a flip or pageboy.

193. What is the best brush for long hair?

Use a large cushion paddle brush like the Curlmaster Paddle Brush. This type of brush provides a larger base on which to brush the hair, thus allowing for more hair to be brushed with each stroke. Large round brushes, like the Phillips Super Round, are excellent for adding waves and curls to long hair.

194. What is the best brush for short, cropped hair?

Use any vent, cushion or small round brush. It depends on what you are most comfortable with and the style you are trying to achieve.

195. What is the best brush for my children's hair?

Children's hair and scalp need extra gentle treatment. Use a very soft bristle brush for children under age 2. Once a child's hair has grown in enough to cover the scalp or reaches the shoulder, use a stronger bristle for brushing the hair. Ball-tipped brushes are also gentle on the scalp.

F.Y. 👁 Haircut How To

- ✂ Chin-length bobs are best for those who don't like frequent cuts and don't need versatility. Five minutes to style. Trim every 6-8 weeks.

- ✂ Medium-length cuts are for women who like long hair and versatility. Twenty minutes to style. Condition weekly. Trim every 6 weeks.

- ✂ Short layers for women who want no-fuss styling and don't mind frequent trims. Five to eight minutes to style. Trim every 4 weeks.

---

196. I am 60-plus and have gray hair. What brush is best for me?

Gray hair is usually more coarse and difficult to style. A stiff bristle brush is recommended, like the Continental WNR21 Oval Cushion Brush or Continental WNR 9000DT Vent Brush.

197. I have a rubber base brush with molded nylon teeth. When should I use it?

Use when styling with a hand-held blow dryer. This brush allows you to brush through wet hair, detangle and style all at the same time. It is especially suited to thick hair. Check out the Denman D3 or Beautique 9-Row Cushion Brush.

198. I am using a wire brush. Could this cause split ends?

Wire brushes without either an epoxy ball-tip or rounded or tapered ends tend to break the ends of the hair because the wire ends are rough and can catch and pull the hair. These types of brushes are also rougher on the scalp. Try using a wire brush with ball-tips or tapered ends, such as the Stance Fanci Multi-Colored Cushion Brush.

199. Should I share my brushes and combs?

Sharing brushes and combs is definitely not recommended for health and hygiene reasons.

200. When should combs be used?

Combs are best used on damp, towel-dried hair for combing through tangles. Combs are also used for sectioning hair, and can also be used on dry, short hair to fix a hairstyle. Wide-toothed combs are best for detangling hair. Basic combs include the Starflight Styling Comb and Rattail Combs.

201. What type of comb should be used on wet hair?

A detangling comb, such as Mebco's small or large detangler, is best for wet hair. Two rows of teeth are positioned to create a detangling effect on the hair. This is a must for long hair. A brush should not be used on wet hair because it can damage it.

202. What kind of comb should be used for "teasing"?

Special combs with small serrated teeth between the longer teeth are used as teasing combs. The smaller teeth on the teasing comb pack hair toward the roots to create fullness and volume in the hair. The best comb for teasing depends on the thickness of hair. For fine, thin hair, use a comb with tightly-spaced teeth to achieve volume and lift, such as Mebco Touch Up or Mebco Little Tease Touch Up. For thicker, coarser hair, a comb with medium to wide-spaced teeth with serrated edges is most effective, such as Comare Mark V Comb, Mebco's The Tease or Mebco Handle Pik.

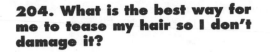

203. Is there a special brush that can be used for teasing the hair?

Yes. It is called a teasing brush, such as the Continental Teasing Brush, which consists of three rows of tufts set in a narrow block with a shaped handle. Use for teasing and lifting hair or creating a sculpted effect.

204. What is the best way for me to tease my hair so I don't damage it?

Use a fine, medium or wide-tooth comb with serrated edges for teasing. Use a narrow-width comb for fine hair, medium-width for medium hair and wide comb for thick hair. To tease hair, do not pull on the hair too tightly. Hold the hair lightly at the ends and gently tease the hair just above the root line. This will add the volume you need to achieve lift. Carefully pick the hair to finish the style. Hair can be teased every day as long as you are gentle. If hair is long, use a teasing brush instead of a comb.

205. What are picks used for?

Picks are used to lift hair for volume and body. They finish a style or build fullness into the style without pulling the curl out. Picks are also great detanglers when hair is wet. Try Mebco's small, medium or large picks.

206. I'd like to try Velcro self-holding rollers, but don't want them to fall out of my hair. Will I need bobby pins?

To properly use Velcro self-holding rollers without bobby pins, first section hair and comb smooth. Press end of hair section gently to roller. Then, roll firmly toward scalp, being sure hair is smooth and even on roller. Press each side of roller against the head to secure. The loops on the rollers grab hair and hold it in place.

207. I have long thick hair, and my Velcro self-holding rollers do not hold my thick hair securely. What can I do?

You may not be using the correct roller size. When rolling hair, use smaller sections and a roller small enough so that hair wraps around the roller completely at least once, yet is large enough so that hair does not wrap more than six times.

208. How can I remove Velcro self-holding rollers without tearing my hair out?

Hold roller by the sides and firmly unroll away from the head. Do not try to pull or slip roller out. Premier self-holding rollers have a single Velcro loop and are more gentle on hair. They cause less breakage and do not tangle as badly as some brands.

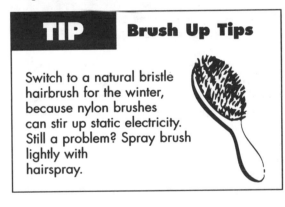

TIP **Brush Up Tips**

Switch to a natural bristle hairbrush for the winter, because nylon brushes can stir up static electricity. Still a problem? Spray brush lightly with hairspray.

209. How do I clean Velcro brand self-holding rollers?

Clean by rubbing two Velcro self-holding rollers together in opposite directions while running under hot water.

210. How should I curl my hair on non-heat rollers when it is dry?

Spray hair with either a spritz or spray gel,

such as Fantasia Ultra High Heat Styling Mist, then roll hair on self-holding rollers and blow dry. Other types of non-heat rollers can be used, but they generally require sitting under a hair dryer or using a bonnet-style hair dryer, which can be attached to your blow dryer.

211. What size roller do I use to get lots of curls if I am using non-heat rollers?

Use small diameter rollers—1/2" size—or pin curls. Apply a firm styling lotion, such as Ion Sculpturing and Designing Lotion, before setting hair.

212. How do I get a smooth, yet full look using non-heat rollers?

Roll using jumbo rollers, such as the 1 1/8" Jumbo Blue, the 1 1/2" Bouffant Red, or 2" Giant Purple Velcro self-holding rollers and blow dry hair. Smooth on just a dab of hair shiner first before rolling.

213. My hair is coarse, curly and thick. What non-heat roller is best for me?

Use a roller that will allow air to flow through the hair to promote faster drying. Self-holding or plastic mesh rollers would work well for you.

214. How many different sizes and types of self-holding rollers are there?

Sally Beauty Supply carries two different types of self-holding rollers—the single loop,

Premier brand, and double loop, Velcro brand, styles. There are 12 different sizes.

215. What are the best rollers to sleep in?

Self-holding rollers, like Velcro rollers or foam cushion rollers.

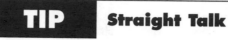 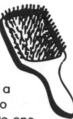

TIP   **Straight Talk**

To straighten coarse, thick, wavy hair by blow drying, hair must be completely blown dry before you try to coax out the curl. When hair is totally dry, use a flat paddle brush that helps to smooth hair strands down. Do one section at a time, using a blow dryer on medium setting and the paddle brush. Start at the back of the head, near the nape. Brush underneath hair, close to the roots, then over the surface for a smooth finish. Try using a light spritz on your brush and going over hair to help hold it.

216. What are flexi-rod curlers, and how do you use them?

Flexi-rods are long cushioned rods which bend in any direction and can be used for setting hair or perming.

217. I like using magnetic rollers. How do they differ from self-holding rollers?

Magnetic rollers are used for wet sets. Magnetics give a smoother and longer lasting

curl because they are usually used on wetter hair. Self-holding rollers are used primarily on dry or slightly damp hair to create soft curls or full-bodied styles.

218. My hair is fine, thin and straight. What is the best non-heat roller for me?

Magnetic rollers are usually the best bet for fine, thin hair because they do not "grab" the hair and there is little chance of breaking the hair. Magnetic rollers come in 13 different sizes to achieve any curl you want.

219. What is the best way to hold my non-heat rollers in place?

Special wire roller pins or double prong roller clips.

220. My hair is short and straight. How do I get wave and curl without a perm?

Use small diameter rollers or pin curls for a curly look, and wave clamps for waves. Use a firm styling lotion before setting hair. Blow dry hair with a diffuser and let cool before brushing.

221. My hair falls flat after I set it on rollers. What's wrong?

You could be rolling your hair improperly or using a roller that is too large for the type of curl you want. To roll hair, hold the hair section at a 45-degree angle from where hair is parted, and roll hair directly back onto the base of the hair strand. Use a styling lotion like Acclaim Plus Setting Lotion or Ion Anti-Frizz Gel Mist.

222. My hair gets the frizzies from rollers. What happens?

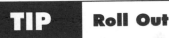

You could be setting your hair on rollers that are too small for the type of curl you are trying to achieve. Also, be sure that each hair strand is combed completely smooth before rolling it onto the roller.

223. After setting my hair on rollers, what is the best way to dry my hair for the most lasting curl?

Using a hot dryer—either convertible-bonnet or hard-bonnet type—will set the curl fastest and give the longest lasting curl. Remember to let curls cool before combing through or you'll weaken the curl formations. The same is true when using a curling iron.

224. I love the look of a French roll. My stylist suggested a ratt. What is it?

Ratts are hair foundations made of a sponge-type material and used to create fullness and sophisticated hair rolls, like the French roll. They can be used on all types of hair, from extra-thick to extra-fine hair. Ratts are made from featherweight foam for comfort and durability. You can even sleep on them! To use a ratt, position the foundation on the hair where you want the roll. Fasten each end of the foundation to the hair with a bobby pin. Push the pin through the foundation or pin over the foundation by squeezing the end.

Smooth hair over the foundation and tuck the ends of hair under the foundation with a comb or brush. Fasten with hair pins. Voila! French roll!

225. I have medium to long hair and would like to wear my hair in a chignon. How do I create this chic look?

Purchase a doughnut-shaped ratt. Pull hair back in a ponytail and pull ponytail through the doughnut hole. Shape hair around the ratt and secure ends under the ratt with hair pins that match your hair color. To hold stray hairs in place, spray lightly with a light hairspray. Tip: If hair is thin, tease hair slightly before shaping around ratt, smoothing hair as you tuck ends under.

TIP   **Roll Out**

Pop in your Velcro brand rollers before hitting the shower. Steam from the shower will set curls. Let hair dry on rollers

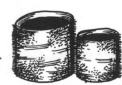

while you dress. When you've finished your makeup, your hair should be ready to comb out and style.

---

226. Should I use hair pins or bobby pins for French twists and chignons? What is the difference?

Hair pins are open at the end and are used to hold large amounts of hair in place. Bobby pins are crimped at the end to hold small amounts of hair tightly. Both are used to cre-

ate the base of support for either a French twist or to hold a chignon ratt in place.

227. How do you set pin curls?

Twist hair, wrap around a finger, then clip in place; or tie two strands of hair together in several knots, then wrap around a finger and clip in place.

228. What styling tools can I use to create Marcel or finger waves?

On damp hair, apply a styling lotion or gel throughout hair, and comb through. Working in sections, push hair gently into desired wave and hold with a wave clamp, either in 3 or 4 inch width. When hair is completely dry, remove clamps. If you want a full look, you can fluff waves with a pick or brush out lightly.

229. I saw rag-tied pincurls in a magazine recently. What are they, and how are they done?

Rag-tied pincurls will produce texture throughout the hair. How much texture depends on the length of hair and where the ties are placed. Reinforced salon cotton coil cut to the needed length works very well for this (try Cellu-Dri Perm Coil in the handy 10 foot bag). Working from a side part, take 2 inch square sections of damp hair. Start 1 inch away from the scalp. Tie coil in a knot around the hair section. Continue tying wherever you want texture. For extra texture, spritz hair with a styling spray like Acclaim Plus Setting Lotion or Spray Gel. Dry hair, remove ties and style with fingers or pick.

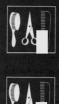

230. What kind of clip should I use for pin curls?

Double or single prong clips.

231. What is the difference between plastic jumbo clips and other clips?

Plastic jumbo clips are larger and have a stronger hold. They are used on large sections of hair and can also double as hair ornaments. They are available in various styles and colors.

232. What are European-style clips, and what are they used for?

These are unbreakable clips designed for pin curls or to secure rollers.

233. What are duck-bill clips, and how are they best used?

These long, slim clips are used to hold sections of hair during styling or cutting.

234. What can I use to hold my bridal headpiece in place?

Combs can be sewn into the headpiece, or use white hair pins or white bobby pins that won't show.

235. What are hair ornaments?

Hair ornaments, also called "hair accessories," are barrettes, clips, pins, bands, bows, beads, etc., used to decorate or hold the hair. Among the more popular types are: banana clips—curved combs connected at one end, and open at the other to fasten and hold the hair; bunsticks—stick and leather hair items that hold the hair in a bun or ponytail, whereby the stick is pushed through the leather and hair to hold it in place; bunwarmers—caged, dome shapes made of metal or plastic that fit over a bun and are held in place with a stick; bobby pins—usually decorated and used to hold hair in place; chopsticks—basic hairsticks resembling chopsticks; ponytail accordian comb—a combination accordian clip and banana comb that gathers up the hair; snoods—a bow with a net on the bottom used to contain a bun or loose hair; spiker comb—a two-piece toothed comb that interlocks in the hair to gather it into a pony tail; twisters—fabric gathered and sewn onto a piece of exposed elastic; as well as classic headbands, ponytail holders, barrettes and bows.

236. I have noticed models wearing a crown of curls on top of their head. How can I create this look if I don't have a lot of hair?

Usually a hairpiece, such as a wiglet or long weft of human hair, is used. The hairpiece is styled prior to pinning onto your own hair, or it may be pinned to the crown of your hair first, and then styled with your own hair.

237. What is the best way to fasten a hairpiece to my own hair?

Secure hairpieces with bobby pins or look for hair extension clips that can be easily sewn into your own hairpiece. Many new hairpieces come with their own clips that "lock" the hairpiece in your hair.

238. Is synthetic or human hair best for hairpieces?

Human hair is best if you wish to wear your hair in different styles, because it can be easily cleaned and restyled. Many human hairpieces can also be permed and colored. Synthetic hair is especially suited to braiding.

239. I want to do something special with my hair. My stylist suggested "hair jewelry." What is it?

Hair jewelry consists of hair beads, charms and gems that are glued or pinned onto the hair. A special hair bonding glue is used that washes easily out of the hair. Jewelry is used for hair decoration, and many up-dos feature it.

240. I have long hair and don't want to cut it, but am extremely bored with my look. Can you offer some easy up 'dos that I could manage at home?

Many of the new hair accessories offer wonderful ways to be creative with your long hair. Try a banana clip to pull back hair, a Spiker, which gathers hair into ponytail, a French Twist Comb, which turns a ponytail into an elegant French twist, or the Wrap 'n Style, a fabric-covered cord that twists to create a sophisticated chignon. Many of these accessories, available at Sally Beauty Supply, come with simple how-to instructions.

241. What is the best hair accessory to pull hair off my face without breaking it?

Use headbands or head wraps, stretchy cloth twisters or terry cloth ponytail holders. Also consider rubbing conditioner or silicone hair shiner onto the covered elastic bands so bands do not break hair.

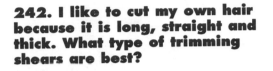

242. I like to cut my own hair because it is long, straight and thick. What type of trimming shears are best?

A shear with one serrated edge, such as the Fromm Sharp Shear, helps to keep the hair in place while being cut rather than pushing the hair away.

243. I have my hair profesionally cut, but often need a quick bang trim to keep me going until my next cut. What type of scissors should I buy?

Select a quality, professional cutting shear with a serrated edge and a 5 1/2 inch blade with finger rest, such as the Fromm Free Cut, the Comfort Grip or the Sheer Glory shear.

244. I have damaged my cutting shears, what should I do?

Most professional shear manufacturers will repair their shears at a nominal fee. Check the warranty card on your shears for the address and phone number.

245. What is the best way to care for my cutting shears?

Always wipe the blades clean and dry after each use. After six or seven uses, place a few drops of clipper or shear oil at the screw points. Always store shears in a dry, safe place.

246. Where do I get my cutting shears serviced?

It is recommended that you return them to the manufacturer for servicing.

TIP   **Short Cuts**

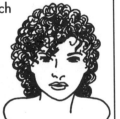

Set short hair on 1/2 inch rollers. Set dry. Then spray with a spray gel or light hairspray. Blow dry with a diffuser and let cool. Remove rollers and sculpt hair into waves with your fingers instead of a brush.

---

247. I have split ends. How often should I have my hair trimmed?

Every four to six weeks.

248. If I have my hair cut every four weeks, will it make my hair grow faster?

No. However, by trimming off any dry, split ends on a regular basis, hair appears healthier.

249. I have a very short haircut and like to keep the nape of my neck trimmed without having to visit my stylist so often. What can I purchase that will allow me to do these quick trims myself?

Use a clipper like the Avanti Clipper Set or the Oster Pro Cordless Trimmer 197-01. Both will help you keep the nape neat between salon visits.

250. When should I use end papers on my hair?

End papers are designed to use on hair that is being permed. End papers may also be used to protect fragile hair when it is being rolled on hot rollers, and are sometimes used on wet sets when hair is rolled on magnetic rollers. They are also helpful in controlling unruly hair that is being set on rollers, particularly when you don't want to risk overuse of gel to control stray ends.

251. Are all salon-quality vinyl capes water and chemical proof?

Yes, if laundered correctly, these capes are water and chemical proof. Be sure to machine wash using cool water. Dry on "fluff" or "air" setting on the dryer. Do not use heat. Chemicals can discolor the cape if not wiped off immediately.

252. I recently purchased special hair clippers. Where can I purchase replacement blades?

Most beauty supply stores, like Sally Beauty Supply, carry replacement blades for most professional clippers, including Andis, Wahl and Oster.

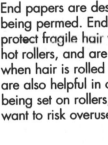

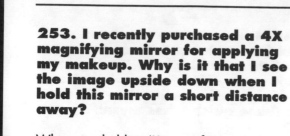

253. I recently purchased a 4X magnifying mirror for applying my makeup. Why is it that I see the image upside down when I hold this mirror a short distance away?

When you hold a 4X magnifying mirror about 18 inches away, you see the image upside down because of the curvature of the mirror. The stronger the magnification, the shorter the distance it takes to turn the image upside down. An image in a 2X magnifying mirror looks upside down at a distance of about 36 inches, twice the 4X mirror.

254. Why are 4X magnifying mirrors not made of glass, but of acrylic?

There are two reasons: cost and weight. The stronger the magnification, the stronger the curvature of the glass needs to be. Using more glass is a difficult process, and it weighs more than acrylic.

255. I love those handy plastic spray bottles. Can I use any liquid in them?

Most are made from sturdy PVC plastic, and any water soluble product, cleaning product, alcohol, disinfectants, water, hairsprays and spritz are fine to use in them. Do not fill them with chlorine bleach products, acetone products, or heavy citrus acid-based products.

TIP Clean Sweep

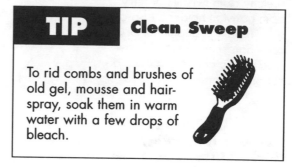

To rid combs and brushes of old gel, mousse and hairspray, soak them in warm water with a few drops of bleach.

Beauty Diary

TOOLS OF THE TRADE

Beauty Diary

TOOLS OF THE TRADE

CHAPTER FIVE

Plug It In

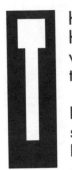

Thomas Edison made it all happen, for without him, women around the world quite probably would still be relying on the sun's rays to dry their hair!

Even before electricity was harnessed, hair was styled with heated implements. As early as 1500 B.C., fire-heated iron bars were used by Assyrian slaves to curl the long tresses of kings, warriors and noblewomen.

The invention of electric hair dryers, blow dryers, curling irons, steam rollers, pressing combs, brushes and crimpers have revolutionized the way women style their hair today. Versatile, time-saving and packable, styling appliances owe much of their invention to two unrelated electrical appliances—the vacuum cleaner and the blender.

During the early 1920s, the idea of blow drying hair originated with vacuum cleaner advertisements proclaiming more than one use of the vacuum cleaner. By hooking a hose to the exhaust of the vacuum, one could easily dry her hair. The idea, however, had a catch. What was needed was a small motor to make the hand-held blow dryer a reality. An appliance that did have a small motor during this time was the electric milk shake mixer and blender, invented in Racine, Wisconsin. In effect, the exhaust of the vacuum was added to the small motor of the blender to produce the modern hair dryer.

Over the next 30 years, the hair dryer was refined with the first major improvement in portable home hair dryers consisting of a hand-held dryer and plastic bonnet that connected to the blower and fit over the head. This $12.95 hair wonder was featured in the 1951 Fall/Winter Sears catalog. Ten years before, beauty legend Jheri Redding invented the first hooded hair dryers for use in hair salons.

Only recently have we seen such an explosion in hair appliance technology. In 1971, Conair was credited with introducing the first pistol-grip blow dryer to the United States, thus signaling the birth of shampoo-and-blow dry hairstyles that revolutionized the way hairdressers and their clients style their hair.

Today, few women (and men) would want to be without their blow dryer, as evidenced by the number of hotel bathrooms which now have blow dryers as standard equipment.

256. What is the difference between professional blow dryers and the "drugstore" variety?

Professional blow dryers have more powerful, longer-lasting motors, which allow for greater air velocity and hotter temperatures. Professional blow dryers are also made from a more durable plastic.

257. What is the most powerful blow dryer on the market today?

The Helen of Troy 1875 Watt Wonderwind blow dryer is currently the most powerful professional blow dryer. Its higher wattage provides more power to dry hair quicker. A special turbo boost button zooms power to 2000 watts.

258. What is the proper way to blow dry hair?

Hair should be towel-dried before blow drying. Use high heat and speed to remove excess moisture from hair. Select lower temperatures and speeds for finishing hairstyles. Lower heat and speeds should be used for drying and styling permed, color-treated or fragile hair. Whenever you brush hair and partly blow dry it against its natural growth pattern, you will add bulk and body to the style. After partially drying hair in this manner, then brush hair and blow dry it in the direction you want your finished style.

259. I travel overseas a lot. What can I do to make my blow dryer and hot curlers work on my trips?

Use a current adaptor and find out what the current is where you will be staying.

Curlmaster and Avanti both make travel dryers that are dual voltage for worldwide use.

260. What should I look for in a travel hair dryer?

A travel dryer should be lightweight, have a handle which folds in for convenient storage, and have dual voltage for worldwide usage. It should have at least two speeds and two heat settings. Curlmaster's 1600 Watt Travel Dryer or Avanti's 1600 Watt Travel Dryer are excellent choices.

F.Y. 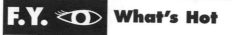 What's Hot

Today's most popular styling appliances are: the hand-held blow dryer, the curling iron, electric rollers, steam rollers, the flat iron or crimping iron, the hot air styling brush, and hair dryers, including the bonnet type which can be attached to a blow dryer. Each do different things.

- Hand-held blow dryers are used to dry wet or damp hair, as well as to style the hair while drying.
- Blow dryers generally are used on high speed and hot settings if hair is very wet; otherwise, low speeds and warm settings are best. They range in power from 1250 watts to as high as 1875 watts.
- Curling irons create individual curls by rolling hair on an electrically heated barrel that varies in diameter from very small (3/8") to jumbo size (1 1/2"). They are often used for touch-ups, spot curls, or all-over curls, and come in two basic types: the spring clamp, which requires only the use of your thumb, or the Marcel iron, which requires the use of the entire hand. The spring iron is much easier to use.
- Electric or hot rollers are heated on a base. Each roller retains heat, and as it cools, it sets the curl. Rollers come in small, medium and large diameters, and are used for spot curls or all over. Hair should cool before brushing to avoid straightening out the curl.
- Steam rollers are sponge rollers held in place by a clamp and heated by steam. As the steam cools, it evaporates and moisturizes the hair. They give hair soft curls and waves which last longer than hot roller sets.
- A flat iron or styling comb straightens curly hair. The very high heat setting is used for straightening and styling coarse, thick, curly hair.
- Crimping irons create a tight, wavy effect. Hair is divided into sections approximately 2 1/2" wide by 3/4" deep. The hair sections are placed between the hot crimping plates and clamped down firmly for two seconds. Hard-to-curl hair takes longer.
- Hot air styling brushes work like a blow dryer and curling iron combined in that warm air is forced through a vented barrel which has "teeth" that grabs the hair as it is curled around the brush. They are used on damp hair to give soft, light curls or wave.
- Hair dryers are used for wet sets, whether they are the salon variety you sit under, or bonnet type that can be attached to your blow dryer. Salon dryers are designed to dry hair faster than the home bonnet variety.

261. My 8 year old insists on her own blow dryer. What would be the best and safest choice for her?

The Avanti 1600 Watt Folding Handle Dryer would be ideal for an 8 year old because it is more compact and lighter weight than traditional hair dryers, yet offers the same features and benefits of the larger size hair dryers.

262. How close should I hold my blow dryer to my hair?

Hold dryer 8 to 10 inches away to remove moisture, and 4 to 6 inches from hair when styling.

263. How long should I dry my hair in rollers under a conventional hair dryer? What setting is safest for hair?

Twenty to forty-five minutes is usually sufficient for drying a roller set, depending on the length of your hair. The setting should never be so high that you are uncomfortable or your scalp burns. It is always safest to dry hair on a lower setting for a longer period than to use a high setting for a short time. Switch to a cool setting for the last five minutes.

264. What is a "cool shot," and how do I use it?

A "cool shot" button on a dryer is a button used to release a "burst" of cool air when pressed while drying hair on any selected speed or heat level. Use the "cool shot" button to direct cool air for a few seconds on a section of hair you are drying to "lock in" the style or curl. Professional dryers with cool shot buttons include Avanti 1600 Watt Turbo and Curlmaster 1600 Watt Turbo.

265. My blow dryer sometimes turns off in the middle of drying. What could be wrong?

First, unplug the dryer and let it cool down. Check the intake vents on the dryer to be sure they are not clogged. You may also be holding the nozzle of the blow dryer too close to the hair. This will also cause the dryer to overheat. Press the reset switch on the safety plug.

TIP   **Cool Tip**

If you've never used a curling iron before, practice with it when it is not plugged in so you won't risk burning yourself. Curling irons are best used to add movement, direction or wave.

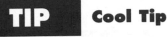

---

266. When using a hair dryer, what heat setting should I use?

A hair dryer should be used on the warm setting most of the time. However, the hot setting should be used sparingly in short bursts when removing excess moisture just after hair has been towel-dried. A hot setting should never be used directly at the roots or scalp. The cool setting should be used at the point at which the hair is dry. Cool air helps set the desired style in place.

267. What setting should I use when I am blow drying my child's hair?

You should always use a low setting of cool to warm when blow drying children's hair. A child's head is very sensitive and their fine hair cannot withstand high heat temperatures.

268. Should you dry your roots only and leave the rest of your hair slightly wet?

No. For best results, dry all of your hair, beginning at the root area and working out toward the end; otherwise, let your hair dry naturally.

269. Do blow dryers damage hair?

No. When used properly, blow dryers will not damage hair. Don't overdry hair. Use the highest heat setting only when hair is very wet.

270. What hair dryers are available that offer a low or cool setting?

Avanti 1600 Watt Turbo Dryer, Curlmaster Turbo 1600 with Cool Shot, Curlmaster 1600 Watt Dryer, and Gold'N Hot Professional Hair Dryers in 1200, 1500 or 1700 wattages are some of the professional dryers available with cool settings.

271. What type of hair dryer is best for someone who does not like to spend a lot of time drying her hair?

Use a high-wattage professional hair dryer since it outputs hotter air. Consider Avanti 1600W Turbo Dryer with Cool Shot, Yellowbird or Blackbird 1600 Watt Dryer, the Curlmaster Turbo 1600 Watt Dryer with Cool Shot, or the Gold'N Hot 1700 Watt Dryer.

272. What is the best type of hair dryer for thin hair?

A dryer with at least two air flow settings as well as various heat settings. For best results, use low air settings and medium heat.

273. My stylist uses a heat lamp to dry my hair. What can I use at home to get the same effect?

A blow dryer with a diffuser attachment will achieve the same effect as a heat lamp.

> **TIP** | **Another Cool Tip**
>
> Professional curling irons are often hotter than those you find in your local drugstore. If you need to cool your professional curling iron down, wipe the barrel of the iron with a damp towel.

274. I have small hands. What blow dryer is best for me?

Many blow dryers have contoured handles designed for any size hand. Look for these handles on the box. Select a medium-size, lightweight dryer, like the Helen of Troy 1600 Watt Mid-Size or Avanti 1600 Watt Compact Turbo Dryer.

275. What should I look for when I buy a blow dryer for everyday use?

For everyday use, your blow dryer should have at least two speed settings and three heat settings. A removable filter for easy cleaning and an 8 foot cord are important features, too.

276. What are those nozzle attachments that came with my blow dryer?

The nozzle attachments are called "air concentrators." They direct the air flow to a smaller area, concentrating the air on one spot.

277. What is a diffuser, and how is it used?

A diffuser is an attachment which fits on the barrel of a blow dryer to disperse the air flow and spread it over a larger area. All diffusers should be used on low speed and cool to warm heat settings. Using a diffuser with a dryer set on high defeats its purpose and can cause the dryer to overheat. A flat-vented diffuser or "finger" diffuser can be used on naturally curly or permed hairstyles. The diffuser dries the curl softly and slowly so the curl pattern is not disturbed. This type of diffuser is excellent for drying straight hair at the roots to add volume and lift. Simply bend at the waist and direct air flow at the nape of the neck and roots of the hair. Keep the dryer moving. Never let the air stay directed at the same spot for any length of time.

278. Which is better, a diffuser with or without "fingers"?

Both are excellent for drying naturally curly or permed hair. A "finger" diffuser can be used to lift and separate the hair, adding volume while drying the hair. It is better for long hair.

Try the Avanti Volume Pik. A flat-vented diffuser achieves the same result, except you need to lift and separate the hair with your free hand while keeping the diffuser in motion over the area being dried. Try the Curlmaster or Helen of Troy Euro Diffuser.

279. What is an easy-to-pack, inexpensive diffuser?

Try the Soft Air Dryer Mit Diffuser or the Soft Diffuse-Aire Diffuser, which fit any hair dryer. Both are especially recommended for naturally curly, permed or wavy hair. Simply slip the dryer mit over the blow dryer nozzle and blow dry hair.

280. Every time I use my hair dryer, I seem to blow away my style. What can I use that will pinpoint one specific area and dry it?

To blow style your hair without hot gusts of air dashing your style, attach the concentrator nozzle on your dryer and use the low speed setting to dry a specific area.

281. Does drying hair under a convertible bonnet dryer take longer than a salon hair dryer?

A salon hair dryer is designed to output a higher air velocity which will dry the hair faster than a home bonnet dryer. Another option for home use is the portable "hard hat" dryer that resembles a salon dryer. Lady Carel offers 1200 watts of drying power, and the Gold'N Hot Hard Hat has a 1200-watt style.

282. Are hoods for drying hair available as attachments for blow dryers?

Yes. There are vented bonnets with an attached hose which connects directly to the barrel of a blow dryer, such as Gold'N Hot Soft Bonnet Dryer Attachment.

283. Are curling irons available with different types of coatings? What is the best type to prevent damage to hair?

There are several different types of coatings. Chrome-plated irons are the most common and most popular, and can be used on all hair types. For thin, fine hair, use on low heat. For medium to coarse hair, use on high. Gold-plated barrels are used on professional curling irons because the gold-plating conducts the heat better, offering higher heat capabilities which most professional stylists require. They are best used on medium to coarse hair. Curling irons with non-stick Teflon™ coating are designed to prevent hair from sticking to the barrel, making them an excellent choice for fine to medium hair.

284. What is the difference between a spring iron and a Marcel iron?

A spring iron has a spring mechanism on the clamp which brings it down and holds it tight to the barrel surface. A Marcel iron has a clamp which is controlled manually by the user, and is most often used by salon professionals. The spring iron is much easier to use because it requires only the use of your thumb to control it.

285. What size and type curling iron is best to achieve a tight curl?

The shorter the hair, the smaller the barrel size needed for a tight curl. The barrel size should increase in relation to the length of hair, up to a 3/4" barrel. Larger than that will not achieve a tight curl. Try the Gold'N Hot 3/8" or the Helen of Troy, Gold'N Hot or Curlmaster 1/2" spring curling iron.

286. What size and type curling iron is best to achieve a wave?

For a wave, a larger barrel size is best. Depending on the length of hair, the 3/4" to 1 1/2" size offers a nice wave. Try the 3/4" spring iron by Curlmaster, the 7/8" or 1" spring iron by Helen of Troy or the Grand Champion 3/4" or 1" spring iron.

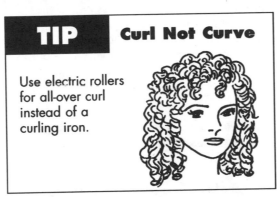

TIP   **Curl Not Curve**

Use electric rollers for all-over curl instead of a curling iron.

287. What is the best way to achieve spiral curls?

Use a 3/4" or smaller barrel curling iron. Roll sections of hair VERTICALLY. When releasing the hair, do not release it all at once. Instead, begin releasing hair at the scalp, or hair closest to the scalp, and slowly unwind by slightly pulling downward. Allow the curl to cool before styling.

288. Can a curling iron be used every day without damaging the hair?

Yes. A curling iron can be used daily on hair without damage as long as you condition hair daily and use styling products which provide thermal protection, such as Keragenics Heat Guard.

289. Which is more damaging to the hair, a curling iron or electric rollers?

Neither is more damaging to hair when used properly. Always follow the manufacturer's instructions.

290. If your hair is not completely dry when you use a curling iron, will it burn your hair?

A curling iron should only be used on completely dry hair because the steam created by the excess moisture combined with the heat from the iron can cause scalp burns. Never use a hot curling iron at roots or scalp.

291. How can I prevent burning myself when using one of the professional 6-setting curling irons?

Practice using your iron at lower heat settings before using higher and hotter settings. When curling hair on these high settings, keep the iron away from the scalp, facial area or other body parts. Do not touch the barrel with your fingers—ouch!

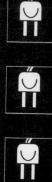

292. I have naturally curly hair that is always out of control. Is there a curling iron available that will straighten my hair without leaving it frizzy?

A large barrel professional curling iron that reaches a higher temperature is best for curly or frizzy hair. Try a 1" barrel for light curl or a larger 1 1/2" or 1 1/4" for super smooth hair. The Gold'N Hot Curling Irons have a rheostat temperature control ranging from 145 to 320 degrees.

293. How soon can I use my hot rollers or curling iron after a perm?

Hot rollers or a curling iron can be used immediately after hair is dry. For fine or fragile hair, wait 24 to 48 hours.

294. Will it damage my hair to use hot rollers after I have had styling products such as gels and hairspray in my hair?

Any thermal styling appliance may cause damage to the hair, whether you have styling products on the hair or not, if special care is not taken to protect the hair and avoid overusing the appliance. Ideally, use hot rollers on clean, freshly dried hair. To prevent damage, use shampoos, conditioners and styling products, like Keragenics Heat Guard, designed to provide thermal protection.

295. What is the difference between a hot air styling brush and a curling iron?

A hot air styling brush works like a blow dryer. Warm air is forced through a vented barrel

which has "teeth" to grab and curl the hair while style drying. Use only on damp hair to finish styling the hair. Hot air styling brushes give soft, light curls or waves. A curling iron does not dry hair like the hot air styling brush can, but it does give hair a tight curl. Helen of Troy makes a hot air brush in 5/8" or 3/4" sizes. Grand Champion offers a jumbo 1 1/2" size.

296. Is a chrome coating or Teflon™ coating better for a curling iron?

Both are equally suited to most hair types, although Teflon's™ non-stick coating is a good choice for fine, thin hair.

TIP **Dryer Double**

Got a spot that you need to get out in a hurry, but can't toss that item in a washer and dryer? Spot-clean dirt and water soluble spots with soap and water. Use your hair dryer on medium-to-cool setting to dry the spot in a jiffy.

---

297. I have gray, thinning hair. Should I use hot rollers or a curling iron?

For everyday use, a curling iron with low heat setting would be your best bet. For curls or waves with added volume, try a steam hair setter, which sets hair without drying it out. Good choices include the Curlmaster Dual Heat Curling Iron, Belson Profiles Steam Express Hairsetter or Caruso Molecular Hairsetter.

298. How should I clean my curling iron?

First, unplug the iron and let it cool down. Use a soft, slightly damp cloth to wipe the surface. Do not allow water or any other liquid to get into the unit. Use a non-abrasive cleaner on the chrome barrel, and baking soda on the Teflon type.

299. I recently purchased a curling iron with 6 settings. How hot will my curling iron get?

The temperature range depends on the type of iron. For example, the Helen of Troy SelecPro Variable Heat Curling Iron heats up to 200 degrees on its highest setting of "10." This iron also offers variable heats to accommodate fine, thin hair to thick, coarse hair.

300. What can I use instead of electric rollers to achieve a quick set?

A curling iron is a good, quick alternative.

301. What is the best size curling iron to use on bangs to curl them back?

Either a 5/8" or 3/4" barrel size are the most effective. They are available by Curlmaster, Grand Champion or Helen of Troy.

 302. What is a flat iron and how is it used?

A "flat" iron or "straightening" iron is used to straighten hair, such as the Gold'N Hot Straightening Iron or Avanti Maxi Heat Iron.

303. How many different brands of flat irons are there?

There are four or five different brands. Belson Gold'N Hot Professional Straightening Iron and Avanti Maxi Heat are two of the better ones.

304. I have naturally curly, thick blonde hair and look like Shirley Temple. What can I use to straighten it?

Use an extra large barrel curling iron, like the Gold'N Hot 1 1/2" size, if hair is short, or a flat iron such as the Avanti Maxi Heat Iron.

305. I have extremely coarse, thick, curly hair. I would like to straighten my hair without using a flat iron. What can I use?

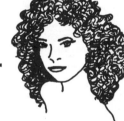

Try a styling comb, such as Belson's Gold'N Hot Styling and Pressing Comb. It has been specially designed to straighten or style very coarse, thick hair. Its variable temperature heat controls provide very high heat for straightening and styling thick, coarse hair, and very low heat for styling extra fine, damaged or dry hair, as well as a full range of heat settings for all normal textures and thicknesses of hair.

306. I like that tight, wavy look, but I don't want to get a perm. What styling appliance should I use?

Try a crimping iron like the Gold'N Hot Crimping Iron. To crimp hair, work with hair sections that are about 2 1/2" wide by 3/4" deep. Place a hair section between the hot crimping plates of the iron and clamp down firmly. Hold in place for only a few seconds. Easy-to-curl hair takes about two seconds to crimp. Hard-to-curl hair will take a little longer. Continue until all sections have been crimped. Hair can be picked out with fingers or styling pick for fullness.

307. What is the difference between steam rollers and hot rollers?

Steam rollers use moisture to lock in curls, while hot rollers use dry heat.

308. Are steam rollers better for your hair than electric hot rollers?

Hair set with steam rollers lasts longer than a style set with hot rollers due to the moisture cooling off the steam rollers. As the moisture cools and evaporates, the curl is set. Two good options are the Caruso Molecular Hairsetter or Belson Profiles Steam Express Hair Setter.

309. Can steam rollers damage color-treated hair?

Steam rollers will not harm color-treated or permed hair.

310. Is there a benefit to using steam rollers?

The benefit in using steam rollers comes from the moisture of the steam. As the steam cools, it evaporates and moisturizes the hair, leaving the hair soft and shiny. The set from steam rollers gives the hair soft curls and waves which tend to last longer than curls from hot rollers.

311. I purchased a Caruso Steam Hairsetter. Where can extra rollers be purchased?

Sally Beauty Supply carries Profile Replacement Steam Rollers which fit the Caruso Steam Hairsetter.

TIP   **Travel Tip**

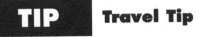

One small wrinkle can spoil a polished look. Blow 'em out with your blow dryer. Using medium-to-high heat, aim your blow dryer at the wrinkle about 8-12 inches from fabric. Be sure fabric can withstand heat. Wrinkle should be gone in seconds! On woolens, spray fabric with a very fine mist of water, then blow dry wrinkles out.

---

312. Why are steam rollers best for thin, flyaway hair?

Steam rollers add moisture to the hair, which adds more volume to fine, thin hair and prevents static which causes flyaway hair.

313. My hair tangles easily. What is the best way to curl easily-tangled hair using a steam hair setter?

Try spraying hair first with a leave-in condition-

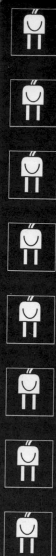

er. When unrolling the rollers, do so slowly, taking care not to pull the roller out of the hair.

314. Will the tap water used in my steam rollers affect my hair?

Tap water used in steam rollers will not affect your hair any more than it normally would. If you live in a hard water area, mineral deposits may build up on your hair. To get rid of this build-up, use a clarifying shampoo like Quantum Clarifying Shampoo.

315. Can steam rollers be used on synthetic hair or wigs?

Yes. Steam rollers can be used on both.

316. How do I clean my steam rollers?

Most steam rollers can be pulled apart by pushing back the foam carefully and sliding the foam off the core of the roller. Clean the foam with a mild detergent in warm water. Rinse thoroughly and blot the excess with a towel. Allow the foam to dry entirely before replacing it on the core for use.

317. I am Asian, and my hair is thick, coarse and straight. Will steam rollers work on my hair?

Yes. If hair is especially hard to curl, consider using a styling product, like Acclaim Plus Setting Lotion, to create a longer lasting curl.

318. How can I create longer lasting curls using steam rollers?

Use a smaller roller with a smaller section of hair, applying more tension when you are wrapping the hair. For extra measure, use a light styling product, such as Ion Anti Frizz Gel Mist.

319. Sometimes I get the frizzies after my hair has been curled on steam rollers. What can I do to prevent this from happening?

Do not oversteam the roller. Follow the manufacturer's directions regarding the amount of time necessary to heat rollers. Be sure to smooth ends of hair on roller when rolling up.

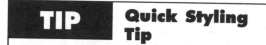

TIP **Quick Styling Tip**

For a quick 'n easy spring or summer 'do for medium-to-long length hair, pull hair back in a ponytail. Pull your bangs (if you have them) forward. Use a curling iron, in small-to-medium barrel diameter, to curl bangs, and to curl several sections of ponytail. Let hair cool thoroughly. Fluff bangs and back of ponytail to create a "mass" of feminine curls. Finish with a firm-hold hairspray. Add a pretty bow or eye-catching hair accessory, and you're ready to go in minutes!

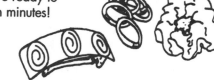

320. Will electric rollers damage my hair?

When used properly, electric rollers will not damage the hair. Always read and follow the manufacturer's instructions. Be sure to let the electric roller cool down before removing rollers so that the curl sets. Removing the curlers before they cool can cause hair to frizz. Using a thermal protective spray like Keragenics Heat Guard prior to rolling gives added protection.

321. What type of hot rollers should be used on thin, flyaway hair? How do I keep them in my hair?

Steam rollers are best for thin, flyaway hair. They are easier to use on thin hair because the hair is held in place on the sponge roller by a clamp which covers the entire curl. Try Belson Profiles Steam Express Hair Setter, or the Caruso Molecular Hairsetter. Try using the 2 to 3 inch wide butterfly clamps on your electric rollers if they slip out.

322. What is the most practical set of hot rollers for someone with short hair?

For short hair, look for a set that has more small and medium size rollers such as Belson Profiles Deluxe Hairsetter with 24 rollers. The hot rollers with raised nobs grip hair best.

323. I have layered hair that is board straight. What is the most practical set of hot rollers for me?

Select a professional roller set that gets extra hot, such as the Belson Profiles Hairsetter, available with 18 or 24 rollers. For curve without lots of curl, try Avanti's Jumbo 1 1/2" Five-Roller Set.

324. I have hair, dirt, dust and spray build-up on my hot rollers. How can I clean them?

Soak the curlers in hot, soapy water, then scrub them with a small brush. Rinse and allow them to dry thoroughly before putting them back on the heating unit.

325. How long should hot rollers heat up before using them?

Most hot rollers have either a "ready dot" on the individual rollers themselves or an indicator light that goes on when rollers are ready to use. Hot rollers are heated on posts which are designed to heat up to a maximum temperature, and then to maintain that level. Rollers should not be left on more than 45 minutes.

326. What direction should I roll my hair on hot rollers?

Roll the hair in the direction you want the curl. Rolling the hair over the top of the roller curls the hair up. Rolling the hair under the roller creates a pageboy style. If the hair is styled back, roll away from the face, if hair is styled forward, roll toward the face.

327. I accidentally knocked my electric rollers into the sink when it was filled with water. Are my rollers ruined?

To prevent the possibility of electric shock, you should not use these rollers again. Say "goodbye" to them and purchase another set for safety's sake.

328. I have a small bathroom and the electrical outlet is above the sink. I'm afraid of dropping my appliances in the sink and shocking myself. Are there appliances that have electric shock protectors?

There are many styling appliances that have automatic shut-off functions in case they are accidentally immersed in water. All professional dryers have this feature, i.e., Gold'N Hot 1700 Watt Dryer, Conair Avanti 1600 Watt Turbo Dryer and Helen of Troy 1600 Watt Dryer with Cold Shot.

329. Will it burn out my curling iron if I leave it plugged in all day by accident?

If it happens only once in a while, the iron should not be damaged. However, to do so continuously risks shortening the life of the iron. Look for a professional curling iron, like The Grand Champion or Avanti Professional Curling

Iron, which will not burn out because they have PTC (positive temperature control) heaters which last five times longer than the standard curling iron heater. As a safety measure, and to prevent any possibility of fire hazard, remember to unplug your curling iron after use.

330. Where can I get my hot rollers and blow dryers repaired?

Contact the manufacturer of the product for their repair. If the item is under warranty, return it to the manufacturer; otherwise, contact the manufacturer to see if they offer repair services or can refer you to someone in your area.

331. Where are replacement blades for electric hair trimmers available?

Check your local Sally Beauty Supply for replacement blades.

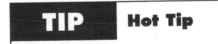

TIP   **Hot Tip**

To prevent split ends, apply a leave-in conditioner or styling lotion to the ends of hair before using a curling iron or hot rollers.

Beauty Diary

CHAPTER SIX

Curl Talk

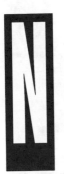

Not everyone was born with curls, but to look back in history at the artifacts, sculptures and masterpiece paintings, one might think otherwise.

Throughout time, curls have been valued for their status, their religious significance, their political message and their sheer appeal.

Men and women have endured the unthinkable simply to have a crown of curls atop their head. Ancient Egyptians heated irons to curl royal beards and wigs. The Greeks used irons and terra cotta rollers. In Rome, the wealthy curled their hair on hollow tubes that were heated by inserting a hot rod. During the Renaissance, "crisping irons" were introduced at the Italian Court. All kinds of contraptions have been used to create temporary curls.

It was not until the early 20th century that a man named Marcel became famous for his way of waving hair in Paris. But it was Charles Nestle who is credited with creating the first permanent wave machine in London in 1905. Nestle's machine involved winding the hair in a spiral on a rod, coating it with an alkaline paste and covering it all with an asbestos tube and a heated gas pipe-iron with tong handles. Electricity was used to heat the large iron clamps while hair was held in place until it had been sufficiently steamed. This method was called croquignole wrapping, and was used primarily on short hair. The entire perm took at least six hours, after which the clients got plenty of curl, and often frizzy, dry, damaged hair with it!

Thankfully, a machineless perm was born in the 1930s, called a "cold wave," now also called an "alkaline wave." In the 1940s, liquid neutralizer was introduced. When perms fell out of fashion in the 1960s because natural looks were "in," acid perms were developed to create softer curls. More recently, conditioners were added to perms to enhance the hair and improve its look.

Today's perms continue to offer many improvements, and there are numerous perms that can be given at home. For best results, see your hair stylist for a professional perm. And, between salon visits, to maintain those glorious curls and wonderful waves, pamper your perm properly!

332. What is the difference between home permanents and professional permanents?

Home perms are usually milder formulas that take longer to process. Professional perms have the advantage of the most current technology and an experienced stylist to help ensure the results.

333. What is a cold wave?

"Cold wave" is a term used for an alkaline wave. This type of perm does not require any added heat to process.

334. What is an exothermic perm?

Exothermic perms contain ingredients that generate their own gentle heat and improve penetration of wave lotion.

335. What is a bisulfate perm?

This is another form of chemical compound that has the potential to curl hair.

336. What is a root perm?

A root perm is used at the root area of the hair only. It is used to perm new growth on the hair that has been previously permed or to add extra lift at the root area. The previously permed ends are protected with products to prevent the waving lotion from penetrating the ends.

337. What is a reverse perm?

A reverse perm is actually the process of taking curl OUT of hair. It can be used to change a naturally tight curl to a looser curl. It is often referred to as straightening hair.

338. What is a spiral perm?

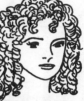

A spiral perm means that shoulder-length or longer hair is rolled onto the perm rod vertically, resulting in a corkscrew-type curl. Spiral perms can also be used to create an explosion of curls. For a traditional perm, hair is rolled horizontally.

339. My stylist suggested I try a weave perm. What is it?

A weave perm waves only part of the hair to provide fullness and curves rather than curl. It is not an easy perm to do, so be sure your stylist is skilled.

340. I have coarse, gray hair. What is the best perm for me?

F.Y. 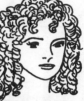 What Makes A Perm Work?

Hair is made of keratin, composed of long molecular chains within the cortex layer of hair. These chains form a twisted rope-like fiber which has a network of cross-bonds or links that provide stability, strength and elasticity to hair. There are two types of bonds: hydrogen bonds and cystine or sulphur bonds. Permanent waves change the hair from straight to wavy by breaking these cross bonds. When hair takes on its new shape, the bonds must be re-established for curl to be permanent.

The classic permanent wave solution or "cold wave" lotion is generally thioglycolic acid plus ammonia, which causes the cystine or sulphur bonds to be released. When hair is wrapped on the rod, this solution is applied. A certain amount of time is required for the hair to take on the shape and size of the rod. This is called "processing time." The stylist must be able to determine how much time is needed to achieve the type of curl desired, otherwise hair can be underprocessed, resulting in curls that relax too soon, or overprocessed, resulting in too curly or frizzy hair. Once the hair is "processed," the stylist applies a neutralizer while hair is still on the rods.

The neutralizer provides a dual chemical action, neutralizing and oxidizing, which results in reforming the cystine bonds and the hydrogen bonds so that the hair stays curled. The neutralizer forms new hydrogen bonds to shrink or harden the cortex and cuticle layers of the hair. The cystine bonds are reformed by oxidation that occurs between the sulphur in the hair and the active oxygen atoms in the neutralizer. When the cystine bonds are reformed, the wave remains permanent. After all the neutralizer penetrates the hair, hair is unwrapped carefully and rinsed thoroughly with water. Now, hair is ready to style.

For best results, perms should be done by a salon professional.

Gray hair is usually very resistant, so your stylist will probably use an alkaline type perm, either a cold perm or an "exothermic" perm. Alkaline perms give a well-defined curl to coarse, resistant hair. An exothermic perm has an extra ingredient that is added to the perm solution and produces a gentle heat during the perming process to give the perm extra strength. There are formulas specifically for gray hair that also have special brighteners to prevent yellowing.

341. Is there a perm on the market that is chemical-free?

No. A perm must have chemicals in it to break the disulfide bonds in the hair and then rearrange them into the new, desired curl pattern.

342. How old should my daughter be before she has her hair permed?

The best age to perm a child's hair is between the ages of 12 and 13 years old because this is the age when the hair has developed its full strength. Perms on younger children usually develop poorly and do not hold in the hair.

343. What is the best type of perm for a child?

An alkaline-based perm is recommended for children. This slightly stronger wave type helps guarantee lasting curls.

344. My new perm is too curly. What can I do to relax it a little?

First, condition hair immediately, then blow-dry hair using a large brush. You may also need to set hair on large rollers. Never use chemical straighteners or relaxers on permed hair because they could damage it.

345. How tight should you pull perm rollers if you want a curly look vs. waves? Does it matter how tight the perm rollers are rolled?

Tension is not a factor to consider when deciding between curly or wavy patterns. Rod size, wrapping techniques and the perm formula chosen determine whether you have curly or wavy hair. Most manufacturers recommend wrapping with minimal tension to avoid damage to the hair. Let your stylist know if you feel the perm rods are wrapped too tightly and are uncomfortable.

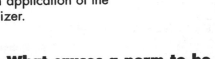

TIP   **Wash Out**

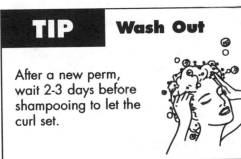

After a new perm, wait 2-3 days before shampooing to let the curl set.

346. What will my hair look like if it is overprocessed?

If hair is excessively curly, hard to comb when wet, fuzzy textured and rough feeling when dry, it has been overprocessed. In extreme cases, the hair is matted, making it very difficult to comb and style.

347. My hair is mushy and looks like cotton candy after my perm. What happened?

Your stylist may have used a wave solution that was too strong, or may have allowed the wave solution to remain on the hair too long.

348. What caused some sections of my permed hair to come out completely straight?

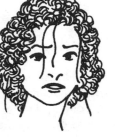

Several factors may cause this: uneven tension while wrapping the rods; loose, but not stable placement of the rod on the scalp; careless application of the wave solution; improper rinsing of the solutions; or uneven application of the neutralizer.

349. What causes a perm to be frizzy?

Usually it is caused by using too much tension when wrapping a perm. Minimal tension should be used so the cuticle can open freely to receive the perm solution.

350. What causes breakage after perming?

This is usually caused by wrapping the perm rods too tight, causing undue stress on the hair while perming, or by placing the perm piks too tightly under the perm rod band, which prevents the hair from expanding naturally during the perm process.

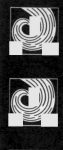

351. I hate my new perm. Can I get it redone immediately?

If you are unhappy with your perm service, go back to your stylist and discuss the alternatives. If it is too curly, it can be relaxed. If it is not curly enough, wait at least a week to redo it. If your hair is not in good enough condition to re-perm, you may have to trim your hair and wait until your hair is ready to perm again.

352. If my perm came out too curly, can I straighten it with a flat iron?

Yes. However, using a flat iron is only a temporary solution. Do not let the flat iron stay on one section of the hair too long or you could damage the hair.

353. I need something to revive my perm. It's only a few weeks old, and it has gone limp. What can I do?

Perm rejuvenators contain moisturizers that add snap to a curl. Avoid heavy conditioners that could weigh hair down. Consult your stylist before the next perm and suggest a different type perm, change of rod size or wrapping technique. Try Quantam Perm Rejuvenator, Design Freedom Perm Revitalizer, or For Perms Only Curl-It-Up.

354. My last perm lasted less than a month. What went wrong?

There are numerous reasons: a bad choice of perm or formula; too much water used during wrapping; not enough water blotted from hair before neutralizing; the stylist missed or skipped a step; hair had excess build-up; a poor consultation, in which the client forgot to tell the stylist something that could have affected the way the perm reacted. Too much or too heavy conditioning during your daily regime can also cause curl to relax. Discuss your problem with your stylist.

355. I'm three months pregnant, and my last perm was five months ago. My hair is a wreck! Can I have it permed now?

Consult you doctor first. Generally, it is safe for a pregnant woman to perm her hair, as long as she doesn't drink the solution! Many stylists recommend waiting until after the first trimester.

356. I like the pageboy look, but my fine, thin hair droops by the end of the day. What perm will give me this sleek look that lasts?

Body waves are perfect for this look, because they'll provide the curve and volume you need to hold your pageboy style.

357. My hair is in that awful growing out stage. What can I do to survive this period?

Let your stylist trim or cut your hair. He or she may also use a spot perm on the new growth. The hair also can be permed on the undersections of the hair to give shape and to make the growing out less noticeable.

358. Can I safely have my hair colored and permed?

Yes. Hair can be safely colored with most types of color and permed, if your stylist uses the correct perm and follows all procedures correctly. However, you may not want to do both processes on the same day. Let your stylist be your guide.

359. Will a perm change my hair color?

A perm should not change your natural hair color. Many perms do fade color-treated hair. Your stylist should rinse hair thoroughly to remove all perm solution from hair to prevent any color fading.

F.Y. 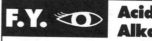 **Acid Or Alkaline?**

There are two basic types of perms, acid and alkaline. Acid perms are the most gentle formulas available. They produce soft, natural, yet long-lasting curls on non-resistant hair. Alkaline perms, also called "cold waves," have more strength and produce a firmer, more resilient curl when used on resistant or hard-to-curl hair types. Exothermic perms are alkaline perms that have heat activators which provide more snap to the curl. New perm technology is producing almost damage-free perms that are ammonia-free and lower in thioglycolic acid. These new perms result in beautiful, springy curls.

360. Why is it important for me to consult with my stylist before I have a perm?

All perms are designed to be used on specific hair types. It is important for your stylist to consult with you first to determine exactly what you want from a perm. It is also important for the stylist to know your lifestyle, medical conditions or time limitations to select the right formula. Then, the stylist must choose the correct wrapping technique and rod size to achieve the results you desire.

361. How do I know if my hair is not too porous to be permed?

Do the "dunk" test by taking a small snip of your hair and immersing it in a glass of water for about 1 minute. If the hair sinks to the bottom of the glass, your hair absorbs moisture too quickly and is too porous to perm. If the hair floats near the surface, it is safe to perm.

362. How long before a wedding should a bride-to-be have a perm?

A bride-to-be should have a perm at least two weeks prior to the wedding so that the stylist can create a look the bride knows she will like.

363. How often is too often to perm my hair?

The normal time period between perms is three to four months for short to medium-length hair as long as hair is trimmed or cut two or three times within this period. Your stylist can help you make this decision.

364. The last perm I had lasted six months. What did my stylist do to make it last so long?

Your stylist chose the correct perm and rod size and correctly performed each step of the perming process.

365. I swim daily in an indoor pool for exercise. Can I have my hair permed?

Yes. If you swim in a pool daily, your hair should be classified as "chemically damaged" because it is being exposed to a high level of alkalinity every day. Your stylist will select the appropriate perm. Be sure to remove chlorine from the hair after swimming with a swimmer's shampoo like Salon Care Anti Chlorine Moisturizing Shampoo.

366. Should I have my hair cut before or after a perm?

Consult with your stylist. Some stylists prefer to cut hair before the perm to remove excess length and weight. Others prefer to cut after the perm to remove any dry or damaged ends and to shape the style.

367. How do I know my hair is in good enough condition to perm?

Your stylist will check to see that you have good elasticity and enough moisture in your hair.

368. My hair is thin, dry and fly-away. Can I have it permed without damaging my hair?

Consult your stylist. Your hair will need extra moisture before perming. A deep moisturizing treatment may be applied to your hair prior to the perm service.

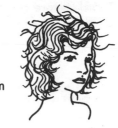

369. Can I go bald from perms?

Perms do not cause baldness. Hair, however, can break off if too much tension is used during the wrapping technique. Also, if the rubber band on the perm rod is twisted, hair can be broken off at the scalp.

370. I get the "greasies" easily. Can I wash my hair after my perm?

If you shampoo immediately after perming, you can relax the curl. Wait at least 48 hours before washing your hair. Until then, wear a hat or pull hair back with a pretty hair accessory.

371. Can I use a blow dryer right after my perm?

You can use a blow dryer after your perm, but it is best to use a low setting and a diffuser. If you brush your hair while drying and pull it straight, you risk relaxing the curl.

372. Is it safe to use a curling iron on hair that has just been permed?

Yes. When using a curling iron, use a thermal protectant on hair, like Keragenics Heat

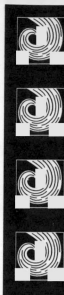

Guard, before curling. Adjust the heat setting to "low" and wind curl. Count to 12 and release iron. Let curl cool before styling.

373. Can I use gel or mousse on my hair immediately after a perm?

Yes. A lighter spray-on gel works well on permed hair. Try Aura Flax Seed Spray-On Gel (flax acts to seal the cuticle). An alcohol-free mousse, like Quantum or Jheri Redding Volumizer, won't dry out curls.

374. How should I treat my hair after I shampoo my new perm?

Gently blot excess water from your hair. Then spray with a light leave-in treatment, like For Perms Only Curl It Up or Ion Anti-Frizz Leave-in, because they won't weigh curls down. Avoid pulling or picking the hair until it is almost dry to avoid breakage and the frizzies.

375. What medications affect the results of a perm? Should I tell my stylist what medicines I am taking?

Always tell your stylist what medications you are taking, and if you have had any recent surgery, including cosmetic or reconstructive surgery. Because medications are excreted through the hair, they could possibly affect the outcome of a perm. Among the types of medications that affect perm results are hormones or high blood pressure medications which tend to make a perm "take" faster than normal. It is believed that these medications raise the temperature of the scalp which accelerates the perm process. Low blood sugar medication can cause early curl relax-

ation. Retin-A can cause the scalp to be more sensitive to chemicals resulting in a burning sensation. Iron supplements can cause the hair to be more resistant to perming. Ask your doctor what effect specific medications may have. It is also a good idea to use a clarifying shampoo before a perm.

376. I work in the sun on weekends. My permed hair is beginning to look parched. What should I do?

If at all possible, wear a hat. Also use styling products with sunscreens, such as Aura, Acclaim Plus or Biotera. Use a daily shampoo and conditioner formulated for permed hair, like For Perms Only Moisturizing or Regular Shampoo and For Perms Only Moisturizer, which add moisture to the hair.

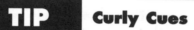

TIP | **Curly Cues**

To keep a perm looking fresh, use professional shampoos and conditioners that are specially formulated for permed hair.

377. Do botanical perms differ from chemical perms? Will they last as long?

All perms contain chemicals in order to work. Botanical perms differ from other types of perms in that they have added botanicals and herbs. Yes, they do last as long!

378. What can I do to get rid of that yucky perm odor in my hair?

There are products available that can be used immediately after a perm to remove residual perm odor. Your stylist should be aware of them. Be sure your stylist rinses your hair longer the next time you have a perm to ensure that all the waving lotion is removed. Many new perms are being introduced that have a more appealing smell. If you are particularly sensitive to perm odor, tell your stylist before having the perm service.

379. Can I have a "cold wave" perm every three months?

It depends on your hair texture and style. Some short cuts will require frequent perming.

380. I had a soft wave at home. When can I have my hair re-permed?

If hair is in good condition, you can re-perm immediately if you want more curl. However, it is best to consult your stylist.

381. How can I cut down on the time I am at the salon for a perm, yet be sure my hair is properly conditioned before the perm service?

Your stylist can use a leave-in conditioner on the hair with some of the new perm products, which not only saves you salon time, but also leaves your hair in excellent condition after the perm. Consult your stylist about using this procedure.

382. My skin burns and sometimes itches while my stylist is perming my hair. What is the reason, and what should my stylist do?

It is possible that your scalp has become pre-sensitized to wave solutions because of the pre-perm treatments. Let your stylist know to give you just one mild pre-perm shampoo and to keep scalp massage to a minimum. Avoid re-conditioning treatments requiring heat.

383. When my stylist was perming my hair, I noticed that purple was running from the hair after he applied the wave lotion. What does this mean?

This is discoloration caused by a metallic deposit, usually iron, in the hair. Minerals are common in hard or well water areas and deposit on the hair during shampooing. Use a clarifying shampoo regularly to help eliminate this mineral build-up on the hair.

384. What is the best size perm rod to get the tightest curl?

The smaller the rod size, the tighter the curl. However, perm formulas provide various strengths and snap to curl. Show your stylist a picture of the style you want so she can determine the best rod size to use.

385. What is a test curl?

During a perm, your stylist will unwind one of the perm rods to check the development of the curl during processing. This test curl should form an "S" shape indicating that the desired curl pattern has been achieved.

386. What is the best size perm rod to achieve waves?

Your stylist will probably use a larger rod size. For very little curl and mostly waves, suggest your stylist use the largest perm rods available.

387. I have fine, medium-texture hair. What is the best perm for me?

Your stylist may use a "cold wave," or a more gentle formulation such as the acid-balanced perm which is heat-activated. This type of perm usually results in soft, loose waves without the risk of frizzies.

388. I want a perm that allows me to wash, dry and go. What type of perm should I request from my stylist?

Your stylist may recommend a curly perm. For best results, your hair should be cut in longer, graduated layers, rather than short layers all over, otherwise you could look like a poodle! The cut is critical.

389. My hair is damaged by sun and chlorine. What perm should my stylist use?

First, you should use a clarifying shampoo to remove the chlorine build-up. Then, consult your stylist regarding whether your hair can be permed. If the sun lightened your hair, a perm for color-treated hair should be used. Your hair may also need moisturizing treatments or conditioning before the perm service.

390. What type of perm should I get for my hair while it is growing out from a perm?

A perm specifically designed for dry or damaged hair would be your best bet. Let your stylist be the guide. He or she may also want to use a moisturizing pre-wrap on your hair to add extra moisture to the dry or damaged areas.

391. My hair falls in my eyes constantly. What perm would help this?

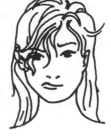

Your stylist would use a directional wrap that forces the hair away from the face and into the desired direction. If your hair is very heavy, you may want to use styling aids to keep the hair in place after you style it.

392. I only want height at the crown. What perm is best for this?

Your stylist would use a spot or root perm.

393. I am of Asian descent with coarse, straight hair. What perm should I have?

Any coarse hair can be permed. Coarse hair is hard to wrap, but not hard to perm. Your stylist would probably use a cold wave and take extra care in wrapping your hair.

394. What conditioning program should I use before my perm?

You should not need a specific conditioning program before perming unless your hair is severely damaged. In this case, consult your stylist.

395. My stylist said he would clarify my hair before perming it. What is this service?

Before perming, your stylist will shampoo your hair with a clarifying shampoo or give you a clarifying treatment to eliminate mineral or styling product build-up on the hair. These clarifying shampoos or treatments used before chemical services like a perm allow the solutions to penetrate more evenly, resulting in a more even curl pattern.

396. What kind of hairspray can I use on my new perm?

Consider using a working spray that easily rinses or brushes out, such as Tresemme 4 + 4 Brush Out Shaping Spray or Ion Hair Spray.

397. I live on the Gulf Coast, and it is so humid my perm frizzes. What can I do?

Use a styling aid to hold hair in place and to seal the cuticle. Use products that contain special humectants and other ingredients to help control the frizzies, such as Ion Anti Frizz Glosser or Frizz Care Hair Treatment. For Perms Only makes a complete line of perm care products which will prolong your perm while reducing the frizzies.

398. After a perm, my hair always looks dull and lighter than its original color. What can I do?

Make sure your stylist is thoroughly rinsing the perm solution from your hair, because applying a neutralizer over the perm solution can cause dryness and lighten hair color. Consider using a shiner on hair, or a color-enhancing shampoo, such as Aura or Clairol Complements, which corresponds to your natural hair color.

399. I love to ski, but when I am in the mountains my permed hair "dies." What can I do to rev it back up?

Try a perm rejuvenator, like Quantum, For Perms Only Curl-It-Up or Design Freedom Perm Revitalizer, to perk up your hair.

400. What special products should I use after I perm my hair?

Permed hair may need extra conditioning. Try Quantum Shampoo and Conditioner for Permed or Color Treated Hair, Keragenics Rejuvenating Treatment and Shampoo or For Perms Only Shampoo and Moisturizer.

401. My hair looks like Shirley Temple—naturally! What products and methods are available to straighten my curls?

Certain wrapping techniques and extra large perm rods can soften curly hair. Chemical relaxers can also be used to straighten naturally curly hair.

402. For a more natural look, what different types of perm rollers should my stylist use?

All perms should look natural. The choice of rod size and type should be discussed with your stylist before wrapping begins. Rod options range from conventional perm rods, spiral rods, and long loop rods to conventional rollers, rags, plastic baggies or cotton coil. The creativity lies with your stylist!

TIP Perm Pick-Me-Up

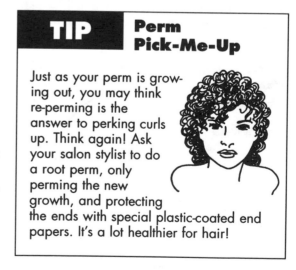

Just as your perm is growing out, you may think re-perming is the answer to perking curls up. Think again! Ask your salon stylist to do a root perm, only perming the new growth, and protecting the ends with special plastic-coated end papers. It's a lot healthier for hair!

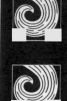

Beauty Diary

CURL TALK

Beauty Diary

CURL TALK

CHAPTER SEVEN

For Women Of Color

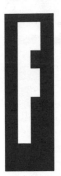

For centuries, African women have regarded curly hair with pride, often decorating it grandly to reflect tribal or family customs.

But when Africans arrived in America as slaves for the wealthy landowners, that once highly regarded curly hair would become a source of both emotional as well as physical pain.

For the next 300 years, blacks in America would endure a myriad of painful processes in an effort to imitate the straight hairstyles of white women.

Hog lard, wagon axle grease, turpentine, kerosene and stove-heated table forks were just a few of the forerunners of today's hair care products designed specifically for the African-American woman.

One person, in particular, is credited with launching the modern black hair care revolution—Madame C. J. Walker. This orphaned daughter of Louisiana ex-slaves built a multi-million dollar hair care business from a single ointment which she concocted on her stove in 1905.

"Madame Walker," as she was to become known in the early 1900s, developed many other hair care products, including an innovative pressing comb that would replace the uncomfortable "pullers" used to straighten hair.

Others followed in her footsteps, like the E. F. Young Manufacturing Co., and Willie L. Morrow, founder of Morrow Unlimited, Inc., who created the cream cold wave for curly hair.

Today, there are many more products than just petroleum jelly and a hot comb to cleanse, curl, straighten and style the characteristically curly hair of women of color.

403. I'm interested in having my hair chemically straightened, but I don't completely understand the process. Exactly what does relaxing involve?

When a woman's hair is relaxed, it is chemically straightened. A relaxer works by penetrating into the cortex and breaking the strong chemical bonds that make hair curly. Relaxing hair begins by protecting the skin around the scalp with a protective cream or oil. A relaxer chemical is then applied to dry hair a section at a time and hair is processed for a specified time. Then, a rinse and neutralizing shampoo is applied to stop the relaxing process. Since relaxing can leave hair in weakened condition, a deep-penetrating treatment is often the final step. A mild straightening solution should be used on fine hair. Hair that is thicker and more coarse can take a stronger solution. For touch ups, a relaxer is applied only to new growth about every six weeks. Relaxers are strong chemicals that are best used by your stylist.

404. I hate the smell from relaxers. How can I minimize this unappealing odor?

Unfortunately, while your hair is being relaxed you can't avoid the odor. However, after relaxing hair, shampooing well with a good neutralizing shampoo, like Sheenique or Isoplus Neutralizing Shampoo, will help remove the odor.

405. If I have coarse hair what would be the best relaxer for me?

A super strength is best for very coarse or resistant hair, and preferably, use a sodium

hydroxide relaxer. See your stylist for the best advice.

406. What is the difference between regular, super and mild relaxer strengths?

The amount of active chemical (sodium hydroxide or calcium hydroxide) determines the strength of the relaxer. Regular is for most people with normal hair, super for very coarse or resistant hair and mild for fine, damaged or over-porous hair.

TIP   **Powder Power**

Powder is a must for black complexions to add warmth, prevent an ashy look and minimize shine. Choose a powder that is close to the foundation shade (which should match skin tone exactly). If the exact shade is not available, try mixing two colors in the palm of your hand to create a good match.

---

407. What is the difference between a relaxer and a curl?

A relaxer straightens the hair while a curl reforms a tight curl into a looser, more manageable curl.

408. What is the difference between lye and no-lye relaxers?

The type of chemicals used. In lye relaxers, the active ingredient is sodium hydroxide. In no-lye relaxers, the active ingredient is calci-

um hydroxide. No-lye relaxer is usually a little milder and good for sensitive scalps, but the calcium can cause hair to be slightly drier.

409. My 10 year old daughter wants her hair relaxed. Is she too young?

Years ago, relaxers for children were not even thought about. In addition to being painful, chemical straighteners used to smell awful, were unpredictable, and carried a high risk of permanent hair and scalp damage. Today, relaxers are much gentler on the hair and scalp and can be controlled. In fact, several manufacturers make chemical straighteners just for children, such as Soft Sheen's Tender Care Relaxer Kit, Proline's Just For Me Relaxer Kit or Lustre's PCJ No-Lye Relaxer Kit.

410. How often can hair be relaxed?

Just like permanent hair color, new growth on hair that's been relaxed needs to be "touched up." This is usually done about every six weeks. The whole head should never be re-relaxed. Relaxing is tougher on the hair than any other chemical process, therefore, only "new growth" should be "touched up."

411. Is there a relaxer for all textures of hair that will not burn my scalp?

No-lye relaxers were developed especially for sensitive scalps. These relaxers are available in a variety of strengths to suit different hair textures. However, if you are extremely sensitive or have dry scalp. Take these precautions:

- Do not scratch the scalp 24 hours prior to relaxing hair.
- Apply a base creme, like Sheenique Scalp Protection Creme, made of petroleum specifically for this use. It also contains menthol and camphor which provides a pleasant, cooling sensation during relaxing.
- Do not apply relaxer immediately after working out or if you have been perspiring heavily. The pores on your scalp are open which can cause a burning sensation during relaxing. To close the pores, rinse hair and scalp with cool water.

412. How can I check for porosity before having my hair relaxed or colored?

To determine if hair has the ability to absorb moisture, take a strand of hair and run it between thumb and index finger of the right hand, from the ends of the hair toward the scalp. If it ruffles or feels bumpy, the hair is porous and can absorb moisture.

413. How can I prevent my hair from breaking at the nape after it has been relaxed?

Hair breakage at the nape of the neck could be a result of pulling hair back too tightly, sleeping in jewelry, wool collars on coats in winter, and most important, improper rinsing and neutralizing during relaxing. Be sure ALL the relaxer has been rinsed and completely shampooed out with a professional quality neutralizing shampoo, such as Revlon's Herbal Deep Clean or Isoplus Upturn Neutralizing Shampoo.

414. Can hair that has been recently pressed be relaxed?

Yes. Pressing the hair is a temporary service which does not affect the cortex of the hair, only the cuticle. However, hair that has been pressed over time can have build-up from the protective oils used with pressing, which can slow down the processing time of the relaxer.

415. How do I know my stylist did not properly roll my relaxed hair?

One of the best ways to tell whether hair has been improperly rolled is if your hair has a "fish hook" at the ends. This indicates that the ends of hair were not properly secured or smoothed around the roller, that hair was unevenly distributed on the roller, or too much hair was rolled on the roller.

416. I relaxed my hair, but as soon as I shampooed it, the curliness came right back. What happened?

The relaxing process may have been stopped too soon. When that happens, it can look like the hair is completely relaxed, but when it is rinsed and shampooed, the natural curl is still there. The process must be correctly timed. Look for instructions that might indicate how long you should wait to shampoo. This could be a contributing factor.

417. How can you prevent over-processing your hair?

Relax, perm or color your hair only when

needed—when there is sufficient NEW growth to warrant the service. When coloring chemically treated hair, use a semi-permanent or long-lasting semi-permanent hair color, which is gentler on processed hair.

418. What are the indications that my hair has been relaxed unevenly?

Frizziness, hair that does not lay flat on the scalp when wet, or uneven curl remaining in sections of the hair all indicate that hair has been relaxed unevenly.

419. How can I prevent that stinging feeling when my hair is being relaxed?

Stinging usually occurs when there is a scratch or abrasion on the scalp or the pores of the scalp are open due to perspiring. To eliminate the discomfort, examine scalp carefully, cool off, and apply a base cream like Sheenique Sensitive Scalp Protection Creme before relaxing.

420. My hair has been recently relaxed, and now has no body. What can I do?

You may have overprocessed your hair. Get hair back on track with a deep-penetrating conditioner, like Ion Effective Care Intensive Therapy which adds protein and moisture. Apply a leave-in treatment after every shampoo and avoid any styling products with alcohol. Try Sheenique Stayz-N Leave On Treatment. Isoplus Unlimited Body Wrap Lotion adds body and bounce to all roller, wrap or blow dry styles.

421. I have relaxed hair. What type of hair regime should I follow?

For relaxed hair, shampoo once a week, use a rinse-out conditioner and a leave-in conditioner twice a week. Use a hairdressing or oil sheen daily. For natural or thermally-styled hair, shampoo once a week, use a leave-in conditioner after shampooing and use a hairdressing or oil sheen daily. For curled hair, shampoo every week to ten days, then use a curl activator every day and curl moisturizer about twice a week.

422. What is meant by the term "overlapping"?

"Overlapping" means to chemically treat hair that has previously been treated. In relaxing or coloring the new growth, care must be taken not to apply chemicals to the previously relaxed or colored hair. A conditioner can be applied to the previously chemically treated hair to prevent hair damage.

423. Can you use a no-lye relaxer over one with lye?

Yes, no-lye relaxer may be used over lye relaxer because the relaxer is always applied to new growth only, not over previously relaxed hair.

424. Can one brand of relaxer be mixed with another brand of relaxer products?

It is not recommended to mix brands.

425. Which section of the head is best to start applying a relaxer?

Start with the most resistant area of the hair, unless you are relaxing hair for a particular design or style. Generally, hair at the nape of the neck is the most resistant.

426. Can I save the unused portion of a relaxer and use it at a later time or day?

All sodium hydroxide relaxers can be saved. Be careful to securely recap the lid after use. Calcium hydroxide or no-lye relaxers should be used or saved only according to manufacturer's directions.

TIP   **Oil Away**

Oil tends to show up easily on black skin. To remedy this dilemma, use a sheer oil-free or water-based foundation. Avoid creamy or thick formulations that tend to look mask-like, and don't forget to carry oil-blotting tissues in your purse to pat away oily shine!

---

427. Is there a relaxer that can remove or loosen natural or chemically induced curls?

Sodium hydroxide or calcium hydroxide relaxers can loosen natural curls. They should never be used on permed curls. Consult your stylist to loosen chemically induced curls. Your stylist will use a permanent wave to loosen those curls.

428. Why is it necessary to use a neutralizing shampoo with a relaxer?

A neutralizing shampoo is used after a relaxer to help remove all traces of the relaxer and help return the hair to its normal pH level.

429. Is conditioning a must for relaxed hair?

Absolutely! Relaxing changes the structure of the hair and can remove some of the keratin protein and moisture from the hair. Condition immediately after relaxing and regularly after shampooing using conditioners, such as Revlon's Liquid Tex Conditioner, Summit Sheenique Reforming Complex, Fantasia IC Reconstructor, Pro-line Perm Repair or Professional Prescription Curative Strengthening Treatment.

430. Will moisturizing my hair cause my hair to go back to its curly shape after it is relaxed?

No. Moisturizing is important to keep hair in tip-top shape—so don't be afraid to do it regularly! Good moisturizing products to try are Ion Moisturizing Treatment, Queen Helene Cholesterol or New Era Hair Moisturizer.

431. What are the best styling products to hold my hair in place after I have just had my hair relaxed?

For roller sets, use a setting lotion, like Revlon Lottabody or Sheenique Bodifi. After drying and styling, keep hair in place with a holding spray, like Isoplus 24 Hour Holding Spray or Sheenique Super Hold Spray. For wrap styles, use a styling gel for maximum hold or a wrapping lotion for softer hold, like Sheenique Freez Hold Styling Gel or Lottabody Wrap 'n

& Tap'n Wrapping Lotion. Follow with a spritz, like Isoplus Upturn Spritz.

432. I don't want to completely straighten my hair. Is there a way to loosen the curl and add texture?

A "texturizing" relaxer or a mild relaxer combed through the hair and left for 19 to 20 minutes will loosen the curl. Kits made specifically for this include Proline's Comb Thru Texturizer, Luster's S-Curl Kit or Duke Texturizing Kit for Men.

433. Does a relaxer curl or straighten hair? What is the difference?

A relaxer is designed to straighten hair. A curl product first relaxes hair, then a waving lotion or booster is used to curl hair. After curling, hair is neutralized like a standard perm would be.

434. What does the statement "patent pending" mean on the relaxer I use?

This term means that either a new ingredient or process relating to the product is new and a patent has been applied for but not issued. The product, however, has passed necessary tests to be marketed.

435. Can African-Americans use any type of perm product?

Yes. Perm products may be used on African-American hair, depending on hair type.

Chemically, a curl product and a conventional alkaline permanent wave have the same active ingredient: ammonium thioglycolate. The difference is that most curl services call for that first "loosening" application of thio (the "rearranger") before applying the waving lotion.

436. Can relaxed hair be chemically curled? Can curled hair be relaxed?

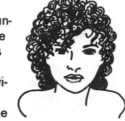

Relaxing and curling cannot be done at the same time. The two processes are different, and the chemicals are incompatible with each other. To do both would break the hair and cause severe damage.

437. What is the safest way to grow out a curly perm?

To grow out a curly perm, keep your hair maintained with curl maintenance products. Wash and condition regularly and moisturize the new growth. For maintenance, try Care Free Curl Hair & Scalp Spray, Wave Nouveau Finishing Mist and Lotion or Right On Curl Activator Moisturizer.

438. Is there a way to curl my hair without using chemicals?

Try roller setting with a body-building product such as Sheenique Bodifi Setting Lotion, Lottabody Setting Lotion or Ultra Sheen Super Setting Lotion. They provide protection and a firmer curl, too!

439. Can I color my relaxed (or curled) hair?

Sure you can! But double-processing is tough on any hair, and double-processing relaxed hair can be especially dangerous. The best recommendation is usually not permanent hair color. Use semi-permanent color instead, or use an "in-between" type color, which doesn't have any "lift," but can last almost as long as permanent hair color. It is best to consult a professional stylist for coloring relaxed or curled hair.

440. How soon after my hair has been relaxed can I have permanent hair color applied?

You should wait 7 to 14 days after relaxing before using permanent hair color. For best results, do a strand test on hair before having hair colored.

441. Can I use henna on my hair?

Regular henna is not recommended for use on hair that has been chemically treated. Ardell's Hennalucent is a 100 percent organic translucent toner and conditioner that can be used on permed or relaxed hair safely. In fact, it will restore elasticity, body and shine as it contains hydrolyzed animal protein, plant extracts and henna.

442. I've always wanted to color my hair red or blonde. Is there a believable shade of red or blonde for me?

There is a shade of red or blonde for everyone! The key is knowing whether you should go red or opt for blonde. Ask yourself what hue your hair turns in the summer. Does it have a red or blonde cast? Use this as a guide to help you find the right shade or consult your stylist. Carson's Dark & Lovely and Soft Sheen's Optimum Care hair color lines are made specifically for African-American hair.

443. Will gray hair be covered by permanent hair color?

Yes. Coverage depends, however, on how resistant gray hair is, the type of color selected, volume of peroxide and proper processing. It is best to consult your professional stylist.

444. How can I be sure the hair color I choose will be flattering to my skin tone?

First, determine your skin tone. Do you have warm (red) or cool (blue) undertones? If you don't know, try this test: try on a white T-shirt, then a beige T-shirt. If the white T-shirt suits your skin color best, your skin has cool undertones. If the beige is more flattering, your skin has warm undertones. Choose hair color with tones compatible with your skin tone. Warm tones are red, gold and auburn. Cool tones are plum, ash and blue. Make a subtle change first. You can always be more daring!

445. Is conditioning important for color-treated hair?

Yes, conditioners seal the hair's surface, returning it to its normal pH level, helping to maintain beautiful, healthy hair. L'Oreal Ineral Hair Fixer can be used immediately after coloring without affecting hair color.

446. How often should I use a conditioner on my color-treated hair?

You should condition color-treated hair every time you shampoo. A leave-in treatment, like Infusium 23 or Summit Sheenique Stayz-N Treatment, will also protect for color-treating. At least once a week, use a rinse out conditioner like Optimum Care Rich Condition, Dark & Lovely Conditioner or Sheenique Nubian Results Conditioner.

447. What is a quick way to remove hair color on my hairline?

Color will remove color. In a pinch, you can take a small amount of hair color from your hair or applicator bottle, add a little water and rub the stain with a soft cloth until the stain is gone. If it's a stubborn dark shade, try rubbing with a little cigarette ash. Also, Roux Clean Touch Stain Remover is a product made specifically to remove color from around the hairline.

448. Will maintenance products affect my hair color results?

Conditioners, scalp creams, styling products, moisturizers, etc., should not affect your hair color. If you have semi-permanent hair color and are using a glycerin based curl activator, your color could fade or run.

449. What will changing my hair color do for me?

Changing one's hair color is one of the quickest ways to get a completely new look. A new hair color can have the effect of making skin look brighter and clearer. It can also give you a psychological and emotional lift. For best results, consult a professional hairstylist when you want to make a major hair color change.

450. If my stylist underprocessed my hair color, how soon can I have him reapply it?

Wait at least 24 hours. This will allow enough time so as to not cause any sensitivity to the scalp area.

451. How do I know which shampoo and conditioner is right for my hair type?

For dry hair, which is brittle, dull and has split ends, opt for a mild shampoo and a deep conditioner with lots of emollients. For damaged hair, which breaks easily, is dry and breaks off when combed, choose a low pH shampoo like Professional Prescription Transpose (5.25 pH) and a deep conditioner, such as Professional Prescription Super Protein Pac or Sheenique Reforming Complex formulated for damaged hair. For excessively oily hair, common among women-of-color with a European or American Indian background, use a shampoo with a higher concentration of detergent than conditioner, such as Revlon Herbal Deep Clean. Opt for an oil-free leave-in conditioner for fine, thin, or delicate hair; hair that lacks body will not hold a set and has static electricity. Select a very mild shampoo, such as Keragenics Therapy or Optimum Care Collagen Moisture and use an instant conditioner, such as Optimum Care Rich Condition or Ion Finishing Rinse.

452. How often should I shampoo and condition my hair?

Every 7 to 10 days is usually often enough—even if you have extensions, cornrows or dreadlocks. If you work out often or wear a wig, you may need to wash your hair more frequently. In this case, a good indication that it's time to shampoo and condition is when your hair begins to look dull, limp or when the scalp begins to itch. Use a conditioning shampoo such as Optimum Care Collagen Shampoo, Summit's Sheenique Silk Moisturizing Shampoo, Revlon's Creme of Nature or Let's Jam Shampoo. Follow with a leave-in conditioner for protection against daily abuse like sun, wind and thermal appliances—Fantasia IC Hair & Scalp Treatment, Sheenique Stayz-N Treatment or All Ways Natural 911 Emergency Treatment.

453. My hair is oily at the scalp but dry on the ends. What do you recommend?

You're describing the natural condition of most African-American hair. The answer is to decide on a maintenance routine—shampoo, conditioner and hairdressing—based on your hair type and how you want it styled. Good products to try are Revlon's Herbal Deep Clean Shampoo or Ion Balanced Cleansing Shampoo along with Ion Moisturizing Treatment or Sheenique Nubian Results Moisturizing Conditioner.

454. What type of shampoo will rinse away heavy doses of hair lotions?

Use a deep cleansing shampoo like Care Free Curl Conditioning Shampoo, Ion Balanced Cleansing Shampoo or Let's Jam Shampoo.

455. What is the best type of shampoo for African-American hair?

Use a non-alkaline, detangling, moisturizing shampoo such as Creme of Nature, Sheenique Silk Moisturizing Shampoo or Optimum Care Collagen Moisture Shampoo.

456. I am an African-American with gray hair. Is there a product that will help reduce the yellow-ish tones?

Try using one of the shampoos designed to reduce yellow or brassy tones in gray hair, such as Jheri Redding Silver Lustre or Clairol's Shimmer Lights.

457. How can I prevent my hair from being dry and brittle?

Shampoo with a moisturizing shampoo like Creme of Nature Detangling Shampoo, Ion Moisturizing Shampoo or Sheenique Moisturizing Shampoo. Follow with a deep-conditioning moisturizing treatment like Ion Moisturizing Treatment, or hot oil treatment like Aphogee Evening Primrose Hot Oil, and a leave-in treatment like Perm Repair Vita-pHlex Leave-in Treatment. Avoid styling products with high levels of alcohol, and use a cream hairdressing daily, like Luster's Pink Oil Moisturizer or Pink Creme Hairdress.

458. My stylist recommended I use a hot oil treatment. What is it, and how do I do it myself?

A treatment using heat and a moisturizing oil

applied to the hair to replace lost oils and moisture is called a "hot oil treatment." Apply oil to hair and cover with plastic. Sit under a warm dryer, use an electric heat cap, or wrap head with hot towels for 20 minutes. Lightly shampoo off with gentle shampoo. Good treatments to try are Sheenique Nubian Silk Oil Treatment, New Era H.O.T. or Aphogee Evening Primrose Hot Oil.

459. My hair is dry, damaged and has broken off. Can I do anything to get it back on track?

It is possible to improve the look, feel and manageability of your abused tresses with conditioners and moisturizers. Try washing hair once a week, using an oil-based shampoo such as Kemi-Moist No-Soap Shampoo and moisturize with a conditioning treatment such as Sheenique Silk Reforming Complex. While the conditioner is in your hair, sit under a dryer for about 10 minutes. Set dryer on moderate to warm heat to allow hair to absorb the nutrients. Also, avoid constant use of hairsprays, or choose one that is oil-based. Brush and comb hair only when needed and be very gentle. Some styling professionals sometimes recommend that their clients with damaged hair have hair extensions or style their hair in cornrows. They're a great way to give your hair a rest while keeping you well-groomed. If you do plan on wearing your hair in cornrows, make sure they are not too tight or left in too long.

460. If I shampoo immediately after my hot oil treatment, am I shampooing out all of the benefits?

No. The heat applied during the treatment opens the hair cuticle to allow conditioning benefits of the oil to penetrate the hair shaft.

461. Can black hair get bleached by the sun?

Yes! Use a leave-in treatment such as Let's Jam Leave-In Treatment that has PABA as a sunscreen ingredient. Also, many finishing products like New Era Oil Sheen Spray and Fantasia's Spritz Hair Spray contain this ingredient.

462. What does castor oil do for hair?

It lubricates and helps promote a healthy scalp. Try Isoplus Castor Oil Conditioner or African Pride Castor & Mink Oil.

463. If I don't want to use an oil-based moisturizer, what can I use to add moisture to my hair?

Try an oil-free leave-in treatment like Ion Anti Frizz Leave-In, Sheenique Stayz-N, Optimum Care Leave-In or Let's Jam Leave-In.

464. Does black hair really benefit from those hot, concentrated conditioning treatments?

Yes. Black hair can benefit greatly from hot conditioning treatments. Because black hair is so fragile and prone to breakage due to frequent thermal and chemical processes, many hair care experts consider them mandatory. Most professionals recommend hot conditioning treatments because heat causes the hair cuticle to open so it can absorb nutrients, vita-

mins, proteins and moisture that have been stripped out of the hair due to any stress.

465. How do I give myself a hot oil treatment at home?

To give yourself a deep conditioning treatment at home, try TCB or Ion Hot Oil, Let's Jam Hot Creme, Ion Effective Care Intensive Treatment or Mend Conditioner. If your hair is truly virgin, use a moisturizing treatment such as Salon Care Cholesterol Conditioner, Ion Moisturizing Treatment and Optimum Care Rich Conditioner. For best results, give yourself a hot oil treatment at home early in the evening to allow the oil to penetrate into the scalp. After washing your hair, apply a very warm—almost hot—conditioning treatment to scalp and hair. After 30 or 45 minutes, wash oil from hair and scalp. Make sure all of the oil is removed.

466. My hair is breaking. What can I do?

Hair breaks because it is weak. Deep-penetrating protein treatments, such as Sheenique Silk Reforming Complex with Silk Amino Acids, TCB Protein Conditioner, Isoplus Deep Conditioner, Proline Perm Repair, can begin to rebuild the strength of the hair's cortex. Use the protein treatment once a week for about a month. Then, to keep hair in good shape, use a professional leave-in conditioner after every shampoo such as Bone Strait Nutri-Shock, Infusium 23 or Sheenique Stayz-N Treatment.

467. Does cutting my hair make it grow more?

No. However, trimming your hair and removing those dry, split ends every four to six weeks will make your hair healthier. Hair grows an average of 1/2 inch per month.

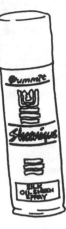

468. What is the difference between a sheen spray and a moisturizing lotion?

Sheen sprays only coat the hair, reflecting light to give an illusion of shine. They provide some measure of protection and make hair easier to comb. Moisturizing lotions adhere to the hair to impart more elasticity and sheen.

469. What is a wrapping lotion, and when should it be used?

Wrapping lotions are conditioning styling lotions that are combed through the hair and molded or "wrapped" around the head to create a smooth style. The head is wrapped with a "wrap cap" and dried. Wrap is removed and hair is ready to go. Wrapping lotions can also be used for blow styling and roller setting. Try Isoplus Wrap Lotion, Lottabody Wrap'N and Tap'N or TCB Bone Strait Wrapping Lotion.

470. How can I keep my hair smooth?

Dab pomade or styling gel, like Sheenique Silk Freez Styling Gel, just around your hairline or braids, then wrap your head with a piece of stretchy fabric or "wrap cap" for 1/2 hour.

471. What kind of pomades can be used to straighten hair?

Pomades cannot actually straighten hair, only make it appear less curly.

472. There are so many hairdressings. How do I know which one is right for me?

It all depends on why you use a hairdressing. If all you want is a healthy sheen, a sheen spray is the best choice. It moisturizes, but does not hold. Lotion from hairdressings moisturize and add some body at the same time. Grease has the consistency of Vaseline, so it can hold sculpted hairstyles. A pomade is the thickest in texture. Examples of some of the many hairdressings available, by type, include: sheen sprays—Isoplus Oil Sheen, Sheenique Oil Sheen and Revlon Finisheen; lotion or creme hairdressings—Luster's Pink Oil Moisturizer, Lustrasilk Moisture Max Lotion and Dark & Lovely Oil Moisturizer Lotion; grease—TCB Hair & Scalp Conditioner, Sheenique Scalp & Root Nourishment, African Pride Herbal Miracle Gro and Allways Natural Indian Hemp Conditioner; and pomades—Sportin' Wave Gel Pomade, Murray's Hair Pomade and Proline Comb-Thru Gel Pomade.

473. My hair has split ends and is very dry and dull. What hairdressing would be best for me?

Use a moisturizing hairdressing to help replace lost oils. Check out Sheenique Herbal Gro, African Pride Castor and Mink Oil or Optimum Care Nourishment.

474. What benefits do botanical ingredients provide in treatment and hairdressing products?

Botanicals provide a wide range of natural benefits, such as cleansing, stimulating, nourishing, refreshing, soothing, moisturizing, normalizing and deodorizing. Chamomile calms, smoothes and adds sheen. Almond moisturizes and cleanses. Peppermint refreshes, stimulates and cools. Flax seed softens and soothes. Aloe heals, restores and moisturizes. Jojoba oil is high in protein to condition and add sheen.

TIP **Eye Appeal**

Eyes can appear tired if the whites take on a yellowish hue. If your eyes deceive you, avoid using brown liner pencils, which can intensify the yellow tinge. Instead, choose eye-brightening colors like gray, black and midnight blue.

---

475. What is a good holding spray with little or no alcohol?

Hairsprays without alcohol generally do not hold as well or dry as fast. However, if you want a low-alcohol hairspray, try Aura Witch Hazel Hair Spray, Resque Alcohol-Free Hair Spray and Ion Anti-Frizz Alcohol Free Hair Spray, which contain no alcohol. However, low alcohol or alcohol-free hairsprays may take longer to dry. Most have similar holding power as those with alcohol.

476. I've worn my hair in cornrows for years, but lately I've noticed the hair around my hairline is getting thinner. What is wrong?

It is possible that your cornrows are pulled back or braided too tightly. Keep cornrows moisturized with a spray made specifically for braids like African Pride's Braid Spray or Sheenique Braid Spray. Stress typically occurs along the hairline and breakage and thinning can occur over time.

477. I use a pomade for shine on my hair, but it makes my hair so stiff. What can I do to get shine without stickiness?

Try a hair shiner for control and shine without stiffness, such as Jheri Redding Replenishing Hair Shiner, Aphogee Gloss Therapy or Sheenique Silk Shiner. For a little more hold with shine, try one of the "ringing gels" like Let's Jam Shining & Conditioning Gel or Bone Strait Shining Gel. (The gel rings when the side of the jar is tapped.)

478. I live in a humid climate and my braided styles tend to frizz. What can I do to help the frizziness?

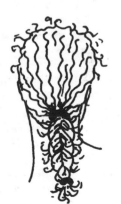

Try a braid spray such as Sheenique Braid Spray or a hair glosser like Ion Anti Frizz Glosser or Aphogee Gloss Therapy.

479. Is there a specific styling aid I should put into my hair prior to braiding?

Try African Pride Braid Spray, Sheenique Nubian Silk Oil Treatment, Kemi Oyl, Let's Jam Conditioning and Shining Gel or Pure Shine Slicking Gel to help make braiding easier.

480. What can I use to help comb through very curly hair that I don't want to relax?

Use a daily hairdressing that is right for you and a rinse-out conditioner after shampooing for detangling. Try Proline Comb-Thru Softener, Liv Creme Hairdress or Optimum Care Light Control Treatment. For detangling, try these rinse-out conditioners: Optimum Care Rich Condition, Ion Moisturizing Treatment, Jheri Redding Humectin Conditioner and Queen Helene Creamy Cholesterol Conditioner.

481. No matter how much pomade, hairspray, gel or mousse I put in my hair it remains dull. What can I use to make my hair shiny?

Applying certain hairstyling products to the hair can add luster. However, too much of a good thing can cause dull hair. For beautiful, shiny hair, shampoo with a deep-cleansing shampoo or clarifying shampoo, such as Care Free Curl Conditioning Shampoo, Ion Balanced Cleansing Shampoo or Ion Clarifying Shampoo to remove build-up. Then, moisturize with a high-protein conditioner and finish by rinsing with cool water. Use styling products sparingly. Try using high-sheen hair glossers, such as Ion Anti-Frizz Glosser, Hask Pure Shine, Let's Jam Oil Free Shine, Sheenique Silk Shine or Aphogee Gloss Therapy. Use just a dab!

482. What gels and hairsprays won't flake?

Higher contents of resin cause gels to flake. Look for a regular hold gel like Sheenique Ultimate Hold Styling Gel, Pre Con Gel Regular Hold or Isoplus Light Styling Gel. In sprays, try Summit Pre Con Spritz, Luster's Pink Oil Holding Spray or Optimum Care Soft Holding Spritz.

483. Can I use styling aids not made especially for black hair? If so, which types?

Yes. You can use most types of styling aids as long as you avoid anything with excessive alcohol or resin content. Try Ion Anti-Frizz Gel Mist, which doesn't contain alcohol. It's crystal clear, won't flake and contains aloe vera for extra protection.

484. I recently had extensions put in my hair. How can I take care of them and my natural hair underneath?

To keep your hair looking beautiful, shampoo every week with a diluted pH-balanced shampoo, being careful not to massage scalp. For best results when shampooing, wet your scalp well before you lather. Rinse well, blot out excess moisture and pat your scalp with a towel. Dry extensions by moving the towel downward. Next, apply a leave-in conditioner. Pat excess with a towel, leaving most of the conditioner in the hair. Then, tie on a cotton scarf and let dry completely. This will help keep extensions or braids looking neat. To prevent flaking or itching, oil the scalp with a natural oil like Sheenique Nubian Silk Braid Oil. Between shampoos, spray on an oil-sheen. Shampoos to try include Ion Balanced Cleansing Shampoo, Sheenique Braid Shampoo and Revlon Herbal Deep Clean Shampoo. For a leave-in conditioner, try Sheenique Stayz-N Treatment or Bone Strait Nutri Shock.

485. I love the latest hairstyles with large French twists, banana rolls and upsweeps. Is there any way I can get my medium-length hair to resemble these styles without investing in a hair weave or buying a wig?

The fastest and easiest way to look like you have hair long enough for many of these popular styles is to purchase a hair ratt. Popular in the 1930s and 1940s, a hair ratt is a lightweight, soft plastic mesh form that comes in several shapes, sizes and colors. To wear one, select a ratt that matches your hair color. Place it where you want your twist. Roll or upsweep hair to cover it, and secure with bobby pins. A dab of styling gel smoothed on will help keep it looking sleek.

486. Which types of combs and brushes are best for African-American hair?

Because your hair is so curly, you want combs made of a top-grade plastic and brushes that you can pull through hair easily, without snagging. Brushes with smooth, pure boar bristles are usually the best choice instead of plastic or nylon bristles that may have rough edges. When selecting a pick, look for wide-toothed types that are coated for extra smoothness.

487. What comb or pick should I use for permed or relaxed hair?

Use a wide-tooth comb or pick, preferably one coated at the tips. Try the versatile "Super Styler" comb with a double-sided comb and a pick on one end. All teeth are dipped to protect from snagging hair.

488. What's the right way to straighten my hair with a hot comb?

The best time to press hair is after you've washed and conditioned it. The hair must be completely dry. Place hot comb in a heater or on a flame. Section hair into several small portions. Apply a pressing oil, such as Sheenique Nubian Silk Oil Treatment or Isoplus Pressing Oil, to the scalp and distribute through the hair evenly and sparingly. Place the hot comb on a tissue paper to test if it's too hot. If the paper scorches, the comb is too hot to use on the hair and should be allowed to cool. Test until the comb leaves no marks on the paper. When the comb is at the right temperature, hold section of hair upward and away from scalp. Pull comb through hair quickly and gently. Make sure hair is touched by the back of the comb (the back rod does the actual pressing). For best results, bring the comb

through each tress twice on top and once on the bottom. Repeat throughout hair. Afterwards, apply a bit of hairdressing to the scalp. Brush through. Comb and style. The Gold'N Hot Pressing Comb has a rheostat that helps take the guesswork out of finding the right temperature. It goes from 145 to 320 degrees.

489. Each morning, I curl my hair with an electric curling iron set on high. Does black hair require very high heat settings?

If you can effectively curl your hair on a lower heat setting, do so. Over time, hot curling damages the hair. Use a protective treatment or styling product which offers some thermal protection, such as Lottabody Setting Lotion, Luster's Pink Oil Sheen Spray or Isoplus Hot, Hot, Hot Curler.

490. Can I use a hot comb on chemically treated hair?

Yes. When using a hot comb on chemically treated hair, it is important to use a lower heat setting and always use a protective leave-in treatment prior to use.

491. I use a heat cap on my hair. What is the temperature range?

The temperature ranges from a low setting of 130 degrees, to medium at 140 degrees, to a high of 150 degrees. Temperatures may vary 5 to 10 degrees. For fine hair, use a lower temperature. Coarse hair requires more heat because the hair shaft is thicker.

492. Will a heat cap dry my hair out?

A heat cap, when used properly according to the manufacturer's instructions, will not dry out the hair. A heat cap should NEVER be used without a conditioner or hot oil treatment.

493. What type of straightening appliance should I use?

Try an electric straightening comb or flat iron such as those by Gold'N Hot. They're convenient and easy to use.

494. What is the best curling iron size to use for black hair?

Size depends on the length of hair, the desired fullness or tightness of curl.

495. What is the best way to dry black hair without taking out the curl or producing frizz?

Use a diffuser and blow dryer, with the temperature set on "cool."

496. On a curl, do I use an activator or moisturizer first?

For a new curl, apply the moisturizer first, which helps combat the drying effect a curl has on hair. Then, follow a program of applying an activator every morning to "activate" the curl pattern while using a moisturizer about twice a week.

497. What can I put on my curl so it doesn't look wet?

Try a lighter formula activator and moisturizer like Wave Nouveau Finishing Mist and Lotion or Care Free Curl Gold Activator.

498. Can people who aren't black use "ethnic products"?

Yes! The use of these products doesn't really have as much to do with a person's race or ethnic origin as the shape and texture of hair. Those with very curly or very coarse hair may only be able to get the styling results they want with a black hair care product.

TIP — Summerproof Hair

Keep sensitive African-American hair from quickly drying out or breaking after repeated exposure to the sun by cutting back on blow drying during summer months. Air dry hair whenever possible, or use a moisturizing cream on hair before blow drying. Work a leave-in conditioner through hair before any lengthy exposure to the sun. Try one with an SPF in it!

CHAPTER EIGHT

Hair Color Cues

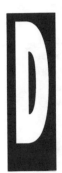

Do blondes have more fun?

While the answer today would most likely be, "Not necessarily," you probably could not convince the fair-haired heroes of Ancient Greece and Rome.

Most Grecian heroes sported light-colored locks, relying on harsh soaps and bleaches from Phoenicia to lighten and redden their hair.

In the 4th century B.C., the Athenian dramatist, Mendener, wrote that the sun's rays were the best means of lightening a man's hair. He described how hair was washed with an ointment made in Athens that turned the hair golden blonde when a man would sit in the sun.

But fair hair was not the color of choice for all societies. The first-century Romans favored dark hair produced by a black dye made of boiled walnuts and leeks. Early Saxon men dyed their hair and beards blue, red, green or orange.

During the era of Elizabeth I, reddish-orange hair was in vogue for men and women. And in the days of French tyrant Marie Antoinette, pastel tresses prevailed. Hair then was heavily powdered in shades of blue, pink, violet, yellow and pure white, with each color having its own heyday.

The first safe commercial hair color was, in fact, born in France in 1909 when French chemist Eugene Schueller created a mixture based on a new chemical, para-phenylenediamine. This concoction became the foundation of his company, the French Harmless Hair Dye Company. The name changed a year later to one of the best-known names in the beauty business, L'Oreal.

What launched the modern-day business of hair color can be attributed to that American innovation, advertising. Thanks to Clairol and its campaign, "Does She or Doesn't She," coloring the hair became commonplace for millions of women, and certainly, the foundation of many salon businesses.

Prior to Clairol's ad campaign, only about seven percent of American women were coloring their hair in 1950. Today, that number has grown to more than 75 percent, and is expected to increase even more as hair coloring improves and becomes less time-consuming and healthier for hair. As more and more women—and men—go gray, hair color could become as common as a haircut!

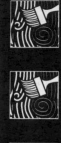

499. What guidelines should be followed in choosing a hair color?

Choose a color close to your natural shade. Consider your skin tone and eye color. Hair color with warm tones, i.e., red, gold and auburn shades, are more compatible with warm skin tones and someone with brown, green or green-hazel eyes. These colors of eyes have the presence of yellow. Cool-tone colors, i.e., lighter gold or ash, are more suitable to fair skinned or sallow skin tones. Eyes are usually light to dark blue or hazel-gray, with no yellow. Make a subtle change first. You can always go more daring the next time!

500. What does the term "semi-permanent" mean?

"Semi-permanent" means the hair color penetrates the hair only slightly. A true semi-permanent lasts only 6 to 8 shampoos and will not completely cover gray unless you use a very dark color. This type of semi-permanent hair color is not mixed with a developer. Long-lasting semi-permanent hair color lasts 25 to 30 shampoos and is mixed with a developer (peroxide), but does not contain ammonia. It can cover gray, but most cannot make hair color lighter.

501. My stylist used a double process on my hair. What is this?

"Double process" means hair was pre-lightened or bleached, then a toner was used to control unwanted red or gold tones.

502. What is the difference between frosting, tipping and streaking?

Frosting involves pulling several fine strands of hair through a "frosting cap" and using bleach to remove the color. Tipping is a process in which only the tip ends of different strands of hair are bleached. Streaking or painting means to apply color or bleach with a color brush, much like painting. These processes are also known as highlighting which can also be done with squares of foil or other material.

503. My hair has a tendency to feel like straw after it has been colored. What can I use to soften it?

Try a post-treatment like Keragenics Rejuvenating Treatment or Aphogee Pro Vitamin Treatment. Post treatments are made to counteract brittle hair and color fading. They are basically leave-in conditioners with extra ingredients to seal the cuticle and lower the hair's pH level to normal after a color service.

504. I have my hair highlighted on a regular basis. The last time I went into the salon and had it highlighted, my ends broke off. What caused this?

Your ends probably broke off because of repeated applications of a high lift tint or bleach on previously lightened ends. Your stylist should use a conditioner to block the ends and only highlight the new growth.

505. If my hair gets wet, will the color wash out of my hair?

No. Semi-permanent and permanent hair color do not wash out like temporary hair color.

506. How can I get a natural look when coloring my gray hair?

F.Y. 👁 Options On Color

Do you want permanent or semi-permanent color? Your stylist is the best person to help you make this selection. However, choosing one type of hair color over another depends on several factors. If you have more than 25 percent gray hair, for example, your stylist may suggest permanent hair color to cover it. If you want your hair lightened, permanent color is generally a "must." Permanent hair color grows out before it washes out! But, if you just want to experiment and try something different, you could try a temporary rinse that would darken blonde hair, or add highlights to darker shades. A temporary rinse lasts until your next shampoo.

For longer lasting color, your stylist may use a semi-permanent hair color, which lasts through at least 6 shampoos. If hair is fragile, or not in tip-top shape, a semi-permanent or in-between color generally will be gentler than permanent hair color. In-between type color is between permanent and semi-permanent. It contains no ammonia and does not lift color, so it is as gentle as semi-permanent color, yet lasts almost as long as permanent color—up to 25 to 30 shampoos. The most stressful process on hair is a double process in which hair is bleached first, then colored.

Choose hair color a shade lighter than your natural color. This will blend better and won't result in that all-one-color look that says, "I dyed it."

507. How do I compromise and still have my hair colored and keep some of the gray?

There are many ways gray can be blended into the hair. Your stylist may color only some strands of hair either darker or lighter, using foil or a cap. You could also try one of the semi-permanent or long-lasting semi-permanent hair colors that blend gray without covering it completely. These hair colors fade naturally with no harsh regrowth.

508. What is color glossing, and how long will it last?

Color glossing is a shimmer of color achieved by using permanent hair color mixed with a developer (peroxide) and conditioner. It is left on the hair a short time, usually 15 minutes. The result is a hint of color and gray masking. It usually lasts for 10 to 15 shampoos. Again, this should be used by a salon professional as the proper shade selection is critical.

509. I am a brunette. Can I have my hair highlighted?

Brunettes can have wonderful highlights. Highlighting can be achieved by applying bleach to those areas where lightness is desired. A powder bleach can be used for this service, as long as it is "off the scalp" work. Another option is to frost or foil highlight with a lightener, resulting in a soft gold. Then overlay the entire head with a long-lasting semi-permanent hair color. Overlay with a color several shades lighter than your natural color. It is best to consult your stylist for highlights.

510. Is henna the only natural plant dye?

Henna is a vegetable-based dye which is made into a paste with water and then applied to the hair to create a strong, red-orange shade that lasts as long as semi-permanent color. Henna coats the hair so thoroughly that it builds up over time, and it can interfere with perming or relaxing, as well as other types of color. Synthetic henna products include Ardell Hennalucent which is compatible with all chemical salon services because it does not coat the hair.

511. What are lead acetate dyes?

There are few successful lead dyes in the professional market. Two common types are Youth Hair and Grecian Formula. These colors are applied frequently to the hair to build up or coat the hair. However, sometimes this adhering process results in "off tones," such as green!

512. My hair has been permed. Is it safe to color it?

Yes. Semi-permanent colors work very well with permed hair. For best results, consult your stylist.

513. Will having my hair colored relax my perm?

Coloring the hair has a negligible effect on your perm. The processes for perming and hair color are different. Perming, however, may affect hair color, and re-coloring the hair after a perm may be necessary.

514. Which does the most damage to hair, a color treatment or a perm?

If products are used as directed, the levels of damage are low and similar for both perms

---

F.Y. 👁 Color Cues

When having hair colored for the first time, your stylist may use some unfamiliar terms. First, he or she will determine the "level" of your hair, which is the depth of your hair color's shade, whether it is light, medium or dark. Levels range from 1 (black hair) to 10 (lightest blonde). Then, the tone must be established, which is the base shade of your hair at the time your hair will be colored. Tones range from warmest red to coolest ash. Tone is an indicator of how warm or cool hair color is, and it is often referred to as the hair's "base color." There are about a half-dozen different tones. When your hair color is "lifted," this means that your natural color is lightened so that the new color can be deposited into the hair shaft. When permanent color is deposited in one step, the process is a one-step or "single process." A "double process" involves first lightening the hair with bleach, which changes the level of the hair color. The second process is applying new color to achieve the new, desired tone. When a color product is used after bleaching it is often called a "toner." Generally, the toner is a permanent color, but semi-permanent and the new "in-between" type of color products can be used as toners, too.

and hair color. Significant damage is due to misuse of the product or errors in processing. Always consult your stylist for best results.

515. What kind of "shelf life" do hair color products have?

Hair colors used to have freshness dates stamped on them. Some still do, but manufacturer testing has shown that the shelf life of hair color is almost unlimited if the bottle has never been opened.

516. Should my stylist save the tint mixture for using on my hair the next time I come in?

Once a hair color has been mixed, it should be used immediately. Any leftover color should be discarded. Your stylist should record the formula used on your hair, the application method and timing of your hair color to ensure you get the same results the next time your hair is colored.

517. My stylist used a new bottle of permanent color on my hair, and I noticed that my hair was a different color than the last time I had my hair colored. What caused this to happen?

Each time you have your hair re-touched, the hair you start with is not the same. It changes due to shampooing, styling, etc. Your stylist may have to check the porosity of your hair before re-touching and alter your hair color formula accordingly.

518. Is there a way to remove permanent hair color?

This is tricky. A color remover is used when artificial color needs to be removed from the hair. It requires more "lift" than either bleaching or a permanent tint can provide. The products that remove the permanent hair color are powerful and can only be purchased and used by a salon professional.

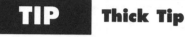

TIP   **Thick Tip**

Permanent hair color can actually make hair seem fuller and does thicken hair strands, but be sure not to go too dark if hair is really thin. Lots of contrast between hair and scalp actually emphasizes thin hair.

519. I hate the color my stylist put on my hair and want to return to my original hair color. What should I do?

Return to your stylist. Depending on whether your new color is lighter or darker than your natural shade, your stylist will do several things. If it is lighter, using a deposit-only color will deepen it. Your stylist would choose a shade slightly lighter and warmer than your natural color to compensate for the higher porosity level in your colored hair. If your hair is too dark, your stylist will use a color remover to lighten the color. After the unwanted color is removed, your stylist will apply a new shade to create the tone you want to return hair to its natural color.

520. What is the least harmful way to color my hair?

Semi-permanent hair colors do not chemically change the hair shaft and are considered to be less damaging to hair than permanent hair color.

521. I am going to have chemotherapy. Can I have my hair colored during the chemotherapy treatment period?

Consider using a semi-permanent or temporary hair color, which are easier on your hair. However, due to the effect of medications and treatments on the outcome of hair color, it is best to consult your physician before having hair colored.

522. What are vegetable glazes?

Vegetable glazes are semi-permanent glazes that provide a slight change of color and last two to six weeks. They give hair shine and body and are usually activated by heat; i.e., 5 to 10 minutes under a dryer produces a temporary color reflection, 15 to 20 minutes offers semi-permanent color and 30 to 45 minutes makes color last six to eight weeks. Glazes, like Ardell's Lights and Brights, can enhance color or just provide healthy shine.

523. I am a brunette and want to lighten my hair with highlights. What should I do about my very dark eyebrows?

Ask your stylist to give you highlights that would complement your natural brow color, so you do not have to lighten them. However, your stylist can also lighten your eyebrows to complement your new hair color. Never try to do this yourself!

524. Can I use permanent hair color on eyelashes and brows?

There are special products designed specifically for coloring eyebrows and lashes. Ask your stylist to color your brows at the time you are having your hair colored. Regular permanent, semi-permanent or in-between type hair color should not be used because they can be very harmful if they get in the eyes.

525. Can hair color be used on a mustache or a beard?

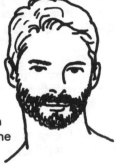

Yes. There are specific hair color products that have directions for use on the beard or mustache. The key is to control the application so that the face is not covered with hair color! For best results, consult a professional stylist.

526. I have a hairpiece that I use for dramatic updos for special occasions. Can my hairpiece be colored to match my new hair color?

If the hairpiece is made of human hair, it can be colored to match your hair. Try the new human hair extension kits with a variety of hair lengths.

527. How often can I color my hair?

Hair can be colored as long as the hair fiber is strong and the scalp is not sensitive. If hair is spongy or breaks easily, use a semi-permanent hair color formulated for damaged hair and begin a rigorous conditioning program. Generally, touch-ups should be done every four to five weeks, depending on the growth of the hair. If you begin to get the "zebra stripe" effect, you know you have waited too long!

528. How do extremely hot or cold temperatures affect hair color?

Most professional hair color products are tested at high as well as reduced temperatures. Prolonged exposure to either extreme, however, may cause the product to deteriorate. If you suspect this, do not use the product.

529. How does hard water affect hair color?

Hard water containing a lot of minerals can discolor the hair or cause it to fade more quickly. Prior to coloring hair, use a shampoo designed to remove mineral deposits, such as Action Environmental Hard Water Shampoo, Quantum Clarifying Shampoo or·AVEC All Pure Shampoo

530. I would like to experiment with a new hair color. What will give me a bit of color, yet not be permanent?

Use a temporary rinse to change the tone of your hair color and to blend gray. You could

try Fancifull Mousse or Rinse, or Wella's Color Charm First Color Temporary Hair Color.

531. What can I expect from temporary color?

Temporary color does not penetrate the cortex. Instead, it coats the outside of the hair shaft so it will wash out in one or two shampoos. Temporary color is great for last-minute touch-ups before a big party or to "make do" between appointments with your stylist.

532. How long does a color rinse last?

A rinse is considered temporary hair color, which means the color does not penetrate the hair shaft. Color rinses generally last only through one to two shampoos. Although there is no chemical reaction, if hair is damaged and porous, the color can penetrate and stain the hair. Be sure to use a color you won't regret!

533. I will be attending a costume party and want to spray my hair gold. What kind of product will not damage my hair, and how can I get the spray out of my hair before going to work the next day?

For special events, use a spray hair color available in an aerosol can. These products come in many colors, including gold and silver. They are temporary colors which come out completely after the first shampoo.

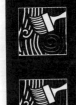

534. I will be going to a costume party and want to temporarily color my hair. What products should I avoid?

Avoid any hair color products made to last through more than one shampoo. Choose, instead, a temporary rinse or hair color spray, like one from Jerome Russell.

535. How long before the wedding should the bride-to-be have her hair colored?

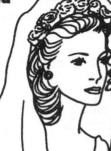

Brides-to-be should experiment with hair color and a perm at least once before the wedding. Since color is performed every six weeks and hair is permed once every three months, a bride needs to decide on a hairstyle, perm and hair color at least three to six months before the wedding. This allows her time to try hair colors and perm styles before the BIG DAY! The stylist will want to practice the hairstyle with the headpiece at least once before the actual event. You should plan to visit the salon at least a week before the wedding for this "rehearsal" so you can enjoy the event, not have a "bad hair" day!

536. I will be doing a lot of television appearances and want to have my hair colored. What should my stylist do so that my hair color appears natural on television under the bright studio lights?

Television studio lights can make hair color look more intense. Red tones are particularly intensified by this type of lighting. Your stylist should keep this in mind in selecting a hair color.

537. In addition to a rinse, what other temporary colors are available?

Colored mousses and color sprays can change a look temporarily.

538. I will be out of the country for several months and not able to have my hair colored. What can I pack that will get me through the "tell tale" gray stage during my trip?

Tuck a temporary rinse or color crayon in your bag. Good ones to try are Fanciful Rinse, Wella's First Color Rinse or Tween Time crayons.

539. My stylist lightened my hair, and it turned out red! What can I do?

Your stylist may choose a new hair color and try again. To neutralize the unwanted red, he or she will use a shade with a blue or green base at the same level. You will probably require a shorter processing time, because the first color application will have increased your hair's porosity. It will be important that your stylist check every minute to ensure the desired results have been achieved. Be sure you consult a professional, as this is no time for amateur hour!

540. I had my hair lightened and don't like it. Can I go back immediately to my original color?

Yes. The trick is, the bleaching has lifted much, if not all, of your natural color. In addition, the color service has increased the porosity of your hair. For these reasons, most color manufacturers recommend using a color filler first. The new color should be one, or even two levels lighter than your natural hair color, because if your hair has been lighter for some time, going back to your "true color" will seem a lot darker than you may remember it. It's safer to go a little lighter for the best overall effect.

541. When my stylist colored my hair, the result came out too dark. Why did this happen?

Your stylist may have selected a shade that was too dark, or the porosity of your hair may have affected the darkness of the color.

542. I am having my hair colored an auburn shade, but do not want an orange halo around my hair line. What can I do?

When coloring hair, many stylists use a chemical buffer in a gel or cream form which keeps the chemicals from running and prevents stains on the skin.

543. I am a brunette and have been coloring my hair. I would like to go auburn, but am concerned about my hair turning orange. How can my stylist prevent this from happening?

Your stylist might try using two parts of a red-orange color and one part of a gold color at a medium brown. Follow with a color-enhancing shampoo for redheads to prevent orange tones from appearing. Try Clairol Complements Color-Enhancing Shampoo or L'Oreal Programme Colour Shampoo in Red Copper.

544. My hair has been permed and colored, but the color is fading and I have dark roots. What can my stylist do that will not dry my hair out, yet will get my color back in shape?

Your stylist can use a permanent hair color on the roots only and match that same color with a semi-permanent color on the rest of the hair. Because hair is more porous on the ends than in the new growth, the semi-permanent color will be more gentle to your hair than the permanent color.

545. About six or eight weeks after I have had my hair colored, my hair begins to turn a lighter shade on the ends. How can I darken the ends of my hair without having my hair completely recolored again?

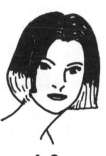

Your stylist could darken the ends of your hair with a long-lasting semi-permanent hair color. This deposits color into hair without lightening the new growth. Choose a shade slightly lighter than what you want, because these colors tend to develop a bit darker on hair that has been previously color-treated.

546. My hair was highlighted too much, and I look like I have white hair. What can I do?

Your stylist can weave low lights through your hair, which involves weaving darker strands through the hair.

547. I would like to go blonde, but do not want to bleach my hair. Is this possible?

That depends on your natural hair color. Black, dark brown or even medium brown hair requires pre-bleaching. Without it, the hair would just turn orange! It is possible to go from light brown to blonde with a "high-lift" tint that lightens up to five levels of color.

548. Is it true women look better as blondes as they get older?

This is a myth. As people age, their skin tone tends to change and lighten. For this reason, a SOFTER hair color rather than lighter hair color is more flattering. While very dark or very bright colors look harsh, a brunette or auburn color can add color and brightness to mature skins. A hair color that is too light can make the skin look washed out.

549. I would like to be a blonde for a day. What is the best way to achieve this?

With today's high-lift tints, just about anything is possible! But just for a day is probably not a wise undertaking. Use a spray-on color, or purchase a blonde wig. If you want permanent color, trust your fate to an experienced professional stylist.

550. I have dark roots, even though my hair is naturally blonde, and I do not want to color my hair. What can be done to blend my dark roots with the rest of my natural hair color?

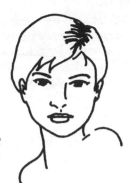

Your stylist can apply large patches of highlighting at the roots to blend them with the rest of your hair. After adding color, each section of hair is wrapped in foil and then exposed to a heat lamp to let the color penetrate. These warm, blonde, color-correcting highlights blend the dark roots into the rest of the hair.

551. I have lighter hair and want to go darker. Will adding permanent color to my already bleached hair damage it?

What you are referring to is professionally called a "tint-back." This is a corrective hair color service which should be done by a professional stylist. Your stylist will also tell you how to maintain the health of your hair.

552. I live in Des Moines and have a wonderful stylist in New York who colors my hair, but I can only have him color it every couple of months. What process can my stylist use so that I am not plagued by those awful dark roots between my New York salon visits?

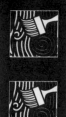

You should ask your stylist about dimensional color. This may be done using foils, a cap, or free hand. By adding highlights on selected pieces, only the harsh regrowth line is eliminated and you can maintain your color every 2 or 3 months.

553. My hair is dark brown and boring! I want to do something different but not drastic. What are some options?

Your stylist can use a double process by first using an all-over gel color to make hair look more vibrant, then applying highlights to achieve a richer, multi-toned look. The result is hair color with depth that looks sun-kissed! This is a complicated process best left to a skilled professional colorist.

554. My dirty-blonde hair is flat and dull-looking. How can I give it some "umph"?

Your hair may need luster, and highlighting can achieve this. Your stylist can apply highlights to thin strands of hair around your face or may opt to do color weaving, which involves applying two different shades of highlights (one slightly lighter than the other). The highlights will last until hair grows out.

555. I have strawberry blonde hair and want to bring out the natural red highlights. What should I do?

To bring out the red highlights in your strawberry blonde hair, simply have your stylist use a semi-permanent hair color in a light blonde level with red tones. Since reds fade more

quickly than other hair shades, maintain your red tone with a color-enhancing shampoo like L'Oreal Programme Colour or Clairol Complements in Red Copper.

556. Where should highlights be applied?

For a subtle effect, highlights are placed on the hair around the face. For a brighter look, apply them throughout the hair.

TIP   **Staying Power**

When having hair colored before going on a long trip, ask your colorist to seal in the color with a special clear, no-color gloss, like Clairol's Jazzing. Color lasts longer and you get great shine.

---

557. Recently, I ran into a long-lost friend whose red hair looked fabulous. However, she was definitely not the same strawberry blonde I knew in school. What did she do to her hair?

She most likely had a single process hair color, because a single process using a permanent or semi-permanent color all over the head produces vivid changes. Generally, for the most dramatic change, the stylist will color hair three shades away from the hair's natural color.

558. I have strawberry blonde hair and want to bring out the natural blonde highlights. How should I do this?

Have your hairdresser apply a lightening product in strands of blonde using a foil process.

559. I'm getting a two-toned effect with my hair color after four weeks. Should hair color last longer than this?

How long hair color lasts depends on how porous the hair is, how much gray it contains, and how fast it grows. The color may fade if the hair is permed or even if you use a shampoo that is too harsh. As a rule, hair should be re-colored before there is more than one-half inch of new growth. Always use a mild, color-safe shampoo like L'Oreal Programme Colour Revitalizing Shampoo, Keragenics Shampoo Therapy or Quantum Shampoo for Permed or Color-Treated Hair. Extend the life of your hair color with a color-enhancing shampoo in a complementing shade as your new hair color. Try Clairol Complements or L'Oreal Programme Colour. For additional protection from color-fading, use a styling product like L'Oreal's Programme Colour Anti-Fading Mist.

560. My hair needs coloring, but is already so dry that I don't want to risk damaging it further. What can I do?

Precondition with a deep-penetrating moisturizing treatment or protein treatment before coloring, like Keragenic's Revitalizing Protein Pac or L'Oreal Programme Colour Treatment Masque. Then, consult your stylist for hair color. Decide what you want the color to do—cover gray, lighten your natural color, lighten selected strands. Pick the appropriate type of coloring, such as semi-permanent to cover gray; permanent hair color to lighten your own color, change its color, and add shine; or highlighting to add dimension and shine without compromising hair strength.

561. Can semi-permanent color be used over permanent hair color?

Generally, you cannot use most semi-permanent hair color over permanent color. The two are designed for different porosities. However, a long-lasting semi-permanent hair color can be used to refresh hair that has been colored with permanent hair color because these colors are created for the same porosity. Be sure to consult your stylist.

562. I've heard lemon juice can be used to lighten hair. Is this true?

Lemon juice is not a good substitute for hair color. It breaks down the hair shaft, literally resulting in a split hair shaft, not just split ends.

563. I am pregnant. Can I have my hair colored?

Hair color is completely safe during pregnancy. However, consult your doctor regarding the effects any medications may have on your hair color.

564. My scalp itches badly when I have my hair colored. What should my stylist do to prevent this?

You could be especially sensitive to the hair color. Your stylist can do a patch test 24 hours before using the hair color to determine if skin is sensitive to the color product. To do this, apply a small bit of color to the inside of the elbow. If redness, itching, swelling or irritation occurs, do not use the product. There are additives for hair color that lessen the burning or irritation of hair color. Your stylist can opt for a gentler product, such as a semi-permanent color.

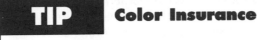

TIP **Color Insurance**

Worried about how styling product build-up may affect your next hair color process? Ask your stylist to use a clarifying shampoo before coloring your hair. And as an added precaution, suggest he or she use a porosity equalizer or a "neutral" color filler to ensure even, natural-looking color.

565. Can two colors be mixed together?

Yes, as long as they are the same type of color, i.e., semi-permanent with semi-permanent or vice versa, and of the same brand. Experimentation with hair color should be left to the professionals.

566. What type of color should be used to cover gray hair?

That depends on how much gray is in the hair. If hair is only 5 to 10 percent gray, a rinse is sufficient, or perhaps a semi-permanent color. For 10 to 25 percent gray, you'll need at least a semi-permanent color or possibly an "in-between" type. If hair is more than 25 percent gray, a permanent color is required for good coverage. Cream colors in tubes have a thicker consistency and often offer somewhat better gray coverage than liquids. Remember, the higher the percentage of gray, the lighter the final color. If hair is one-third or more gray, some colorists recommend mixing in some of the next deeper level of the same tone to achieve the desired results. If you want to simply blend, rather than cover gray, this can be achieved by coloring the hair a level or even two lighter, which creates natural-looking highlights. This will also require less touching up. For best results, consult your stylist.

567. What is the reason for a purple/violet color shampoo for blonde, gray, white or highlighted hair?

Violet shampoos counteract unwanted yellow tones in blonde, gray, white or highlighted hair.

568. What can I do about the brassy yellow tinge to my gray hair?

"Brassy" is a tough term to describe. This yellowish or orange tone looks unflatteringly harsh and has many causes, including over-exposure to the sun, wind or saltwater. Your stylist may use a permanent or semi-permanent color product to neutralize the yellow. This is usually one with a violet base, or possibly a blue base if the brassy tone is more orange, and at the same level as your natural color. The simplest solution may be to use a blue or violet-based highlighting shampoo to neutralize the brassiness, such as Shimmer Lights or Aura Blue Malva.

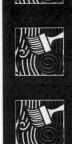

569. What do I use to get the green out of my hair?

Usually a green cast means hair was over-porous or so fine that it grabbed too much of an ash (green-based) color. You must neutralize the green with the color that is opposite it on the color wheel, i.e., red neutralizes green and vice versa. Your stylist will choose a different shade with a red or red-orange base. The new color should be at the same level as the existing color.

570. Does the temperature of the water I use to wash/rinse my hair affect how long my hair color will last?

Use warm-to-tepid water to rinse the hair to protect your hair color.

571. My hair color is fading. How can I boost the color?

Use a color-enhancing shampoo which is designed to freshen or tone the hair. Try Clairol Complements color-enhancing shampoos or Aura Shampoos—Camomile for blondes, Clove for brunettes, Madder Root for redheads, Black Malva for black hair and Blue Malva for gray or platinum hair.

572. Is there a hair color product that also acts as a conditioner?

Most hair color products today contain conditioning ingredients, especially semi-permanent, long-lasting semi-permanent and deposit-only hair color. Hair feels softer and shinier than it did before coloring.

573. I have very blonde hair and want to use a color-enhancing shampoo that will be compatible with my current color, yet work with the darker shade I would like to be. What color-enhancing shampoo will work best for me?

For best results, deepen your hair color with a non-ammonia hair color that deposits color. A color-enhancing shampoo like Clairol Complements will keep your final color brighter.

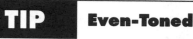

TIP — Even-Toned

When you're trying to grow out your natural hair color, avoid the two-toned stage by asking your stylist to use a semi-permanent color that is one shade darker than your natural color.

574. How do color-enhancing shampoos work?

Color-enhancing shampoos contain dyes that deliver more color the more you use them. They work by building a color reservoir on the cuticle layer of the hair.

575. Can I use color-enhancing shampoos on my child's hair?

Color-enhancing shampoos are gentle enough for use on children's hair.

576. Why can't I see any noticeable color difference after using a color-enhancing shampoo the first time?

You may have selected a shade that is too light. However, color-enhancing shampoos are formulated to emphasize the natural highlights of your hair or to help maintain the brightness and tone of color-treated hair. They are not designed to cover gray or lighten natural hair color. If you want a more noticeable change, consider having your hair professionally colored.

577. If I leave the color-enhancing shampoo on my hair for a longer period of time, will the color be stronger?

It is possible to enhance the effects of a color-enhancing shampoo by leaving it on longer than directions indicate. The amount of color depends on your own hair's porosity at the time you use the shampoo. The more porous the hair, the stronger the color.

578. Do I still need to color my hair if I use a color-enhancing shampoo?

Color-enhancing shampoos work best on hair that has been previously colored because the hair is more porous, thereby allowing the color in the shampoo to more easily deposit on the hair shaft.

579. If I do not like the color-enhancing shampoo I am using, can I switch to another one?

If you would like to try a different shade,

simply use a clear shampoo for a few days, then switch to a new shade of color-enhancing shampoo.

580. Can I mix different color-enhancing shampoos to create a unique shade for myself?

If you are adventuresome, feel free to mix different shades of color-enhancing shampoos. Most color-enhancing shampoos are formulated to be mixable.

581. Will color-enhancing shampoos stain my skin or fingernails?

Some color-enhancing shampoos may stain skin or fingernails. Washing your hands with soap and water or using some hand cream helps remove any stains.

582. I have a marble shower. Will the color-enhancing shampoo stain my shower?

No, staining should not occur.

583. What do I do if my color-enhancing shampoo stains my tub, tile, grout or bath towels?

Bleaching is the most effective way to remove these stains. It may take several applications to totally remove the stain. However, most color-enhancing shampoos should not stain your tub or tile.

584. Why should I do a test patch before using a color-enhancing shampoo?

All hair color products are required by law to state on the packaging that a patch test should be done prior to use. Color-enhancing shampoos are considered a hair color product and contain ingredients that may cause an allergic reaction on some individuals.

585. In the summer, my hair lightens naturally under the sun. What can I use in the winter to lighten my hair like this?

Lightener products developed as gentle lighteners are recommended. Try Sun Go Lightly Maximum Strength.

586. What hair color product will make my hair shine without damaging it?

Ardell's Lights and Brights is a natural product that will add subtle highlights and lots of shine.

587. I love my new hair color. What can my stylist do that will help lengthen the time my new color lasts?

Many stylists will apply a clear color gloss over the hair, such as Clairol Jazzing, which not only helps to further seal the cuticle, but also extends the life of your new hair color. These glosses can be semi-permanent when used with heat or temporary without heat. They are actually very healthy for color-treated hair because they leave hair shiny, and can tone down intensity or modify color on porous hair.

588. My hair grows so fast that a week after my color was put on my gray roots started showing.

What's the quick solution?

For spot retouching, try hair color crayons. They are moistened and applied directly to the roots or hair line, then blended. They work like lipstick for your hair! Best bets are Tween Time Crayon by Roux or Cover That Gray.

589. Whenever I have my hair colored, I end up getting the hair color under my fingernails. What will remove this dark stain?

Stain removers, such as Roux's Clean Touch, will remove stains under your nails or around the hairline. You can also use a product for the nails called Gena "Nail Brite"

590. Why is my new hair color different than what my stylist showed me on the hair color chart?

The color samples are designed to give you an idea of how the color would look on white hair, since about 80 percent of people color their hair to cover gray. Gray hair is a mixture of one's original color and hair that's gone white. The final new color should be at the same level as the existing color.

591. Are hair color products tested on animals?

Clairol and L'Oreal do not perform animal tests with any of its products, either within the company or at outside testing labs. Information required for products can be developed using controlled human tests. For new raw materials, including hair color dyes, testing to provide required safety data may include animal testing.

Beauty Diary

HAIR COLOR CUES

CHAPTER NINE

Nail It

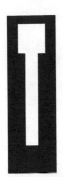

The art of well-manicured nails can be traced as far back as 4,000 years ago in southern Babylonia where the well-groomed noblemen of that time used solid gold implements to manicure their fingers and toenails.

Fingernail polish, however, is believed to have been invented by the Chinese by 3,000 B.C. as a means of indicating one's social status. A 15th century Ming Dynasty manuscript describes how the royal colors for fingernails were black and red.

Egyptians, too, indulged in the art of manicuring and coloring the fingernails, with red being the most important color of social rank. Queen Nefertiti painted her fingernails and toenails ruby red, although Cleopatra, that early beauty queen, preferred a deep russet. Even men painted their nails. It was common for military commanders of ancient Rome and Egypt to have their nails painted to match their lips before they dashed off to the latest battle.

Today, well-manicured nails are as much a part of good grooming as brushing one's teeth or combing the hair. Thanks to modern technology and continual improvements within the nail care industry, the art of manicuring can be at the finger tips of almost everyone!

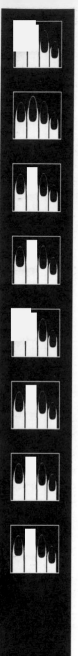

592. How do I maintain great looking hands?

For natural nails, the basic routine should include a cuticle oil or cream and a professional nail strengthening treatment. It's a good idea to have a medium and fine grit file. If you wear polish, you'll need a basecoat, topcoat, polish remover, polish dryer and professional formula nail polish. If you don't wear polish, use a nail buffer to maintain natural shine. You can also treat yourself to a manicure soak, a hot oil treatment or a paraffin wrap. If you choose to extend your nail length with tips, wraps, gels or sculptured nails, use products containing botanical oils to moisturize hands and nails. Avoid products containing mineral oils, since they can cause nail extensions to lift. Basic items for nail grooming include: Contours Botanical Nail Oil, Beauty Secrets Dual Treatment Kit, Beauty Secrets Cushion White Files in medium or fine grit and Beauty Secrets Nail Enamel Dryer Spray.

593. How often should I get a professional manicure?

This depends on your lifestyle and preference. If you prefer absolutely perfect, medium to long nails every day, you'll need a professional manicure once a week. If you favor shorter length nails for an active lifestyle, and you can do polish touch-ups at home, you may need a professional manicure only every two weeks. The faster your nails grow and the more abuse they withstand, the more often you'll need professional maintenance. Apply a protective topcoat every two to three days, like Beauty Secrets Dual Treatment, Orly's Top 2 Bottom or Nail Selectives Radiant Top Coat, to maintain your manicure.

594. What products are available for home use to maintain a professional manicure?

There are literally hundreds of products. For nail strengthening, try Beauty Secrets Nail Hardener and Thickener or L'Oreal's Mighty Nails. To condition cuticles, try Contours Botanical Oil or Beauty Secrets Cuticle Oil. For basecoats and topcoats, try Brucci Base Coat, Nail Selectives Hydra-Coat Base Coat or Nail Selectives Radiant Top Coat. Professional nail polishes from Nail Savvy, Nina or Revlon often last longer than the "drugstore" variety. To remove polish, try Beauty Secrets Acetone, Non-Acetone or Adios Acetone or Non-Acetone polish removers. Dry polish with Nail Selectives Rush Polish Dry/Topcoat, Ultra Set Nail Polish Drying System, Varoom or Beauty Secrets Nail Enamel Dryer Spray. Add nail buffers and nail files, and you're set to keep those nails looking nifty!

595. How long should a professional manicure last?

Generally, a professional manicure will last from one to two weeks, depending on how fast your nails grow and what you do. The faster they grow and the more abuse they withstand, the more often you'll need professional maintenance.

596. Should I give my nails a "breather" between manicures?

The idea of leaving nails unpolished for a few days to let them rest is a common myth. Fingernails are made of dead skin cells, and they don't need to breathe.

597. Is it better to touch up my nail polish between manicures or completely remove all the polish to re-polish?

It's easier and more convenient to touch up the polish on the free edge of your nails between manicures. A manicure always looks fresher if you have the time to completely remove the polish and re-apply fresh basecoat, polish and topcoat.

F.Y. 👁 Facts About Formaldehyde

Formaldehyde is found in a surprising number of things we use every day—even clothing! Most nail polishes and many nail strengtheners contain formaldehyde because it helps polish adhere better, and it is very effective at penetrating and hardening the nail plate. A very small percentage of people experience an allergic reaction to formaldehyde after repeated use. Over time, it can have a drying effect on anyone's nails, which is one more reason to moisturize and nourish with a cuticle conditioner regularly. The U.S. Food and Drug Administration allows the use of formaldehyde in nail care products, but limits the amount permitted to only five percent. If you are concerned about possible sensitivity, look for formaldehyde-free polishes and nail treatments. In general, if it's not overused, formaldehyde has no harmful effects on nails.

598. Is it essential to have nails manicured in a salon?

It is not essential to have a professional manicure, but it is certainly beneficial in more ways than one! Most salon atmospheres are clean, efficient and offer a luxury we all crave—pampering! Treating yourself to a day, or even an hour, at a salon is a refreshing, revitalizing experience. With today's industry standards for salon sanitation and advances in salon technology, the salon is the best environment for nail services.

599. How can I give myself a salon-perfect manicure at home?

A salon-perfect manicure can only be given by a trained professional. To approximate a professional manicure at home, follow these steps: Begin by removing any old polish and cleaning the hands and nails with a nail scrub. Trim and file the nails to the approximate desired length, and shape with nail scissors or clippers and medium to fine grit files. Soften the cuticles with a manicure soak and push them back with a cuticle pusher. Moisturize and nourish cuticles with a cuticle cream or oil. If you wear polish, use one coat of basecoat, two coats of polish and one coat of topcoat polish dryer. If you don't wear polish, use a nail buffer to smooth small ridges and maintain natural shine.

600. The smell of many nail products really bothers me. What can I do about this awful odor?

Be certain to read the manufacturer's directions completely before using any product. Almost all products state they must be used in well-ventilated areas only. Look for products available that have low-odor or are odorless.

601. What would be the best manicure machine to purchase?

The Nail Genie Jr. is perfect for home or travel. It's battery-operated and contains five different attachments to speed up manicures or pedicures.

602. What are the advantages of using an electric or a battery-operated manicure machine?

They speed up the filing, shaping and buffing process.

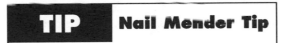

TIP Nail Mender Tip

If you've split or torn a nail and have no mending tape, repair your nail with nail glue and a piece of tea bag or coffee filter paper. Cover the tear and dot on glue; let dry, then file to smooth.

603. I need new attachments for a manicure machine given to me as a gift several years ago. Where can I find them?

Sally Beauty Supply carries replacement attachments that fit most machines.

604. I have scraggly cuticles. How can I get them back in shape?

Massage cuticle cream, oil or lotion into the cuticle. Then, use a cuticle stick to gently push back the cuticle after you have softened it, which in most cases eliminates the need to trim the cuticle. If necessary, cuticle trimming should be left to the professional, who will use special stainless steel cuticle trimmers available in different "jaw" sizes. Best bets are Tweezerman "Pushy" Cuticle Pusher, Winning Nails Plastic Cuticle Pusher, Flowery Thin Manicure Sticks and Tweezerman Cuticle Scissors.

605. If I trim my cuticles will they grow back faster?

Leave cuticle trimming to a professional nail technician. Instead of trimming the cuticles, condition them daily with Contours Botanical Oil or Hoof and Nail Therapy and push the cuticles back. This should help control growth and prevent hangnails.

606. I have half-moons on my nails. What are these?

The technical term for this is the "lunula." The light color of the lunula, also known as the "half moon," is caused by the reflection of light where the matrix (also known as the mother of the nail, where nail growth begins) and the connective tissue of the nail bed join.

607. What is the best way to remove hangnails?

Nail technicians remove hangnails with cuticle nippers. The best way to prevent hangnails is to use cuticle cream, oil or lotion that is massaged into the cuticle and nail mantle. Then use a cuticle stick to gently push back the cuticle after you have softened it, which in most cases, eliminates the need to trim cuticles of hangnails.

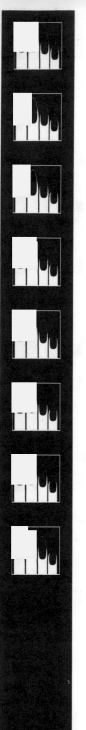

608. My manicurist accidentally nipped my cuticle with her cuticle clippers, and my cuticle started to bleed. What should she or I have done immediately?

The nail service should be stopped immediately. The cut should be cleaned out with an antiseptic and pressure should be applied to the cut if the bleeding continues. Your nail technician should not continue the service until the bleeding has stopped.

609. My cuticle nippers have tightened up so much that I can no longer use them. What will make them usable again?

Oil the hinges.

610. I have a nail biting problem. What product do you suggest I try as a deterrent?

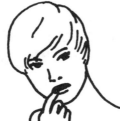

Try having acrylic caps applied to your nails. This type of hard coating may help prevent biting your nails. A liquid product you can apply to your nails to help stop biting is Bite No More by Super Nail.

611. I was a chronic nail biter, but have stopped. My habit has made my cuticles uneven. Is there anything I can do to even out my cuticles?

Have regular manicures, including cuticle cream, oil or lotion that is massaged into the cuticle and mantle. Then use a cuticle stick to gently push back the cuticle. To condition the cuticles, try Gena Healthy Hoof Nail Treatment.

612. I am a nail biter and I have heard that my nails grow faster than most people. Why don't I notice this?

Yes, your nails do grow faster. The reason you don't notice this growth is because you are always biting your nails. Nails grow faster when they are bitten since this a form of stimulation to the nails. To stop biting your nails, try having them coated with an acrylic or something that is almost impossible to bite off. Then you'll notice how fast your nails grow. Also try Bite No More by Super Nail, which is a simple liquid application.

613. What causes puffy cuticles?

Puffy cuticles can be caused by several things. If the cuticle has been scraped, or there are abrasions on the cuticle and chemicals are then used, the skin could be irritated. Puffy cuticles can also be caused by an allergic reaction to products used on the nails or products in which the hands are being soaked. Your professional nail technician can best diagnose the reason for your puffy cuticles and assist with treatment. Professional application of nail products is the best prevention for skin irritation.

614. My cuticles seem to peel after a professional manicure. What can I use to prevent this?

When cuticles peel between manicures, this generally indicates extra dry skin. By regularly massaging cuticle oils and conditioners into the base of the cuticle area, you can help prevent problems like this. Best bets are Contours Botanical Oil, Beauty Secrets Nail Matrix Fortifier or Gena Tea Tree Oil.

615. I have ragged cuticles which sometimes start to bleed when my manicurist files my nails too close to the cuticle. Is it safe for her to apply acrylic on those nails that have damaged cuticles?

Anytime there is blood during a nail service the service should be stopped immediately until the bleeding has stopped. With acrylic nails, the monomer, which is the liquid, should never be applied to the skin. It should only be used as a part of the application on the natural nail.

616. What can I use to keep my cuticles from growing so fast?

Cuticle trimming should be left to the professional, who uses special stainless steel cuticle trimmers available in different "jaw" sizes. However, you can massage Varoom Lemon Brite Cuticle Remover, Adios Creamy Cuticle Remover or Beauty Secrets Alpha Hydroxy Cuticle Remover into the cuticle and mantle, and use a cuticle stick to gently push back the cuticle.

617. What is the most important product that I should buy to keep my cuticles in shape?

There are two types of cuticle oils and conditioners that can be used. Cuticle conditioners that contain mineral oil, should only be used on natural nails to soften the cuticles and prevent hangnails. Cuticle conditioners that contain botanical oils can be used on all nails, including nail extensions, to soften cuticles and prevent hangnails. Try Contours Botanical Nail Oil or Beauty Secrets Nail Matrix Fortifier. Cuticle conditioners that contain mineral oil should never be used with nail extensions because they may cause lifting.

618. There are so many types of nail files. How do I know which one to use?

Choose your file depending on how you plan to use it. The higher the grit number, the smoother the file. Coarse files (80-100 grit) are best for acrylic extensions. Medium files (180 grit) are best to shape extensions of medium thickness, like most tips and wraps, and to shape the free edge of natural nails. Fine files (240-600 grit) are best for removing small bumps, ridges or discoloration and shaping the free edge on the natural nail. (See Chart)

619. My nails are very thick and difficult to shape. Is there anything I can use to thin them?

The best solution for shaping thick nails is to use a medium grit file on the free edge. Frequently, thick nails also have ridges. Natural nail buffers (fine grit) can be used to reduce ridges on the nail surface for the appearance of a thin, smooth natural nail.

620. What is a circular nail disk?

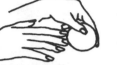

The circular nail disk, commonly referred to as the Round Buffer or Disk File, is used in different ways, determined by the grits of the file. A higher number grit (or a softer buffer) may be used on the surface of the natural nail and nail extensions. The curve of the round disk buffer helps to prevent scraping the cuticle and allows for a natural filing motion on the surface of the nail. A lower number grit (or a coarser file) may be used on the surface of nail extensions with extra care. Both round buffers can be folded in half to file the underside of a tip for

better adhesion. Tropical Shine makes circular nail disks in blue (medium grit), pink (fine grit) and black (combo grits).

621. How do I use a small, four-sided nail board?

The four-section nail buffing board can be used on both nail extensions and natural nails. Begin with the most coarse section, which is usually black or blue. Finish with the smoothest section, which is usually gray. This buffer removes imperfections in the nail and buffs to a smooth, glossy shine. Try Tropical Shine 4-in-1 Buffer or Les Mirage Glas Sheen Buffer

622. Is it better to use a metal file or an emery board?

Either type can be used to shape the free edge of the fingernail by filing corner-to-center in one direction. Never file from side-to-side on a natural nail. This may weaken the stress points of the free edge. A metal file or emery board should not be used on the surface of a natural nail because these files are usually too coarse. Metal files, in general, tend to cause nail splitting. Choose a professional non-metal file like those from Tropical Shine.

623. How should I use a nail buffer?

A natural chamois skin buffer is used with a buffing creme like Winning Nails. For buffers, try Perfect Nails Chamois Stik or Winning Nails Chamois Buffer. Apply a small amount of buffing creme to nail and buff in one direction crosswise on the nail. Rinse and dry nails.

HOW TO SELECT THE RIGHT NAIL FILE		
GRIT	**USE ON**	**USED FOR**
Coarse (80-100)	Sculptured Nails and Tips (Never use on wraps, gels or natural nails)	Removing Bulk or Taking Down Length
Medium (180)	Tips Sculptured Nails Gels & Wraps Natural Nails	Blending Seams Shaping Shaping Filing & Shaping
Fine (240-600)	All Types of Nails	Finishing
Ultra Fine (600-2400)	All Types of Nails	Buffing, Shining

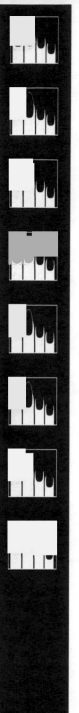

624. Is there any special type of nail file that can be used on nails that are soft?

A fine grit nail file (240 grit) is excellent for shaping the free edge of soft nails or as the first step in removing scratches, ridges or imperfections from the natural nail surface with a three or four-sided buffer.

625. Can an electric filing machine be used on acrylic nails?

An electric filing machine is commonly referred to as a nail drill. Yes, it can be used on acrylic nails. Nail drills are best used by a professional nail technician who has been properly trained to use them.

626. If I shape my natural nails by filing the corners of the nails round, will it make the corners of my natural nails stronger and less likely to split?

The shaping or the filing of the sides of your nails does not make them stronger or less likely to split. If you have a snag on the side of your nail and you do not file it, the nail will tear off. Use the right type of file in a correct fashion. To shape or file the natural nail, you should use a medium to extra fine grit file (180-240 grit). File the natural nail from the corner of the nail to the center of the nail. Never file in a see-saw motion. File the sides of the nail straight and file the end of the free edge to the desired shape. Try Beauty Secrets cushion files in medium to extra fine.

627. What is the best nail length for someone with short fingers?

Nail length is not necessarily determined by the shape or length of the fingers. People with short fingers normally have shorter nail beds, so a medium-to-short length for natural nails if best. If nail extensions are preferred, a shorter to medium length extension is best because nails that are too long on a short nail bed will not be well-balanced with the length of the nail bed and free edge.

TIP **Chip Tip**

After applying topcoat to nails, hold brush parallel to tip of nail and sweep topcoat slightly under nail to prevent pesky chipping!

---

628. I have big, athletic hands. What is the best nail length for me?

People with larger hands normally have medium-to-large nail beds, so a medium length for natural nails is best unless a very active lifestyle requires a shorter length. If nail extensions are preferred, depending on lifestyle, a short-to-medium length extension is best. Most nail extensions work best at a short-to-medium length. Nail tips now come in a variety of lengths and styles to suit all lifestyles and preferences.

629. What is the best nail length for a bride-to-be?

That depends on personal preference and lifestyle. On this very special day, you tend to be hard on your nails. With little or no time for maintenance, a shorter or medium length nail is preferable.

630. I have nail ridges. What causes this problem and can it be fixed?

There are many different causes of nail ridges. Trauma to the nail, certain medications taken over long periods of time, and chronic health conditions can cause temporary or permanent nail ridges. If ridges are temporary, they will grow out within six months to a year. Use nail strengthens and ridge fillers as well as cuticle softeners to promote healthy new growth. If the ridges are permanent, continuous use of a natural nail buffer or chamois skin buffer and buffing cream, like Winning Nails, as well as a ridge filler, like Beauty Secrets Ridge Filler, Brucci Ridge Filler or Nail Selectives Silkfill Ridgefiller, will smooth the appearance.

631. I recently slammed my finger in the car door. As a result, I have a bumpy nail and the nail bed is very sensitive. Will this eventually heal on its own or is there a product to improve the look of the nail or speed up the healing?

The nail will eventually heal on its own. In the meantime, buff the surface of the nail with a natural nail buffer, like Tropical Shine's 3-Way Nail Buffer in three sizes, and use a ridge filler, like Orly Ridge Filler, L'Oreal's Zero Ridges or Beauty Secrets Ridge Filler, to conceal the bump in the nail until it grows out.

632. Why are there white spots on my natural nails?

As a child, you may have been told these were called "lie spots." The more lies you told the more white spots you would have on your nails. This, and all other tall tales, are not true. White spots are calcium deposits in the nail, usually caused by hitting the nail or smashing the nail in a door.

633. Can I use a topcoat as a basecoat or vice versa?

It is best not to use them interchangeably. Although they look similar, these two products are designed to do different things. Basecoats are usually thicker and stickier, which helps the nail polish adhere better. They contain more resins to give the nail added strength. Topcoats are thinner and contain more ingredients that create a durable surface on the nail. They are made to add strength, dry quickly and protect the polish from daily wear and tear. There are a few timesaving combination basecoat/topcoats on the market, such as Orly Top 2 Bottom.

634. Can all fast-finish nail products be used as a basecoat?

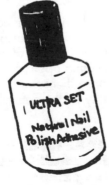

Avoid using the fast-finish nail product as a basecoat unless it has been specifically designed to work as both a basecoat and a topcoat. Most of the fast-finish nail products are not sticky enough to work well as a basecoat. A good basecoat is a little thicker than a top-coat and sticky enough to create a base for your nail polish to adhere. A new, thinner basecoat that resembles a white glue is available for natural nails called "Natural Nail

Polish Adhesive by Ultra Set." Also try European Secrets Molecular Stix—both should be applied very thin.

635. Recently, all my nail polish peeled off in one large piece after a professional manicure. What caused this, and how can I prevent this from occurring?

It is very unusual for polish to peel like this. This may be due to oil or creme applied to the nail and not rinsed off, the basecoat and polish were not compatible or a quick-dry polish that looked like a basecoat was used instead of a basecoat.

636. What is a nail strengthener?

Strengthening treatments are also called nail hardeners, and they are formulated to strengthen the nail plate. The nail plate is made of keratin, the same protein as hair. Some strengtheners actually penetrate into the nail plate to strengthen nails from the inside. These strengtheners often contain formaldehyde to penetrate and harden nails. Protein strengtheners work in a similar way and contain a protein such as collagen. Other hardeners, like a liquid wrap, work on the surface of the nail plate. They contain tiny fibers of a fabric, like nylon, to coat nails for extra thickness. Nail vitamins can always be used in addition to your manicure routine. Nail strengthening treatments to try include Beauty Secrets Nail Hardener and Thickener, Brucci Miracle Formaldehyde-Free Nail Hardener, SuperNail Fiber Nail Wrap (liquid wrap) and Windsor Nail Nutrition Tablets (vitamins).

637. Will rubbing gelatin on my nails strengthen my natural nails?

Rubbing gelatin topically on natural nails to strengthen them is a myth. Nails are dead and can only be nourished from the matrix of the nail or internally.

638. Will using calcium on the surface of my nails strengthen my natural nails?

Using a topcoat containing calcium provides a stronger protective coating to the nails. Try Orly Calcium Shield Nail Builder.

639. How can I make my nails grow stronger?

This is actually asking for two different things. Making the nails grow is only accomplished with the increase of blood circulation or stimulation. Making the nails stronger can be accomplished by using products with moisturizers (conditioners) or proteins. Tips: Massage Contours Botanical Oil into the nail matrix and cuticle regularly to strengthen nails. To stimulate circulation, soak nails in Revlon's Aromasoak using warm water for a great sensory experience.

640. How do I get my nails to grow faster?

There is no "sure thing" to make nails grow faster. The average adult's nails grow one-eighth of an inch per month. Nail vitamins, cuticle conditioners and nail strengtheners all can help promote healthy, new growth. Consider using Windsor Nail Vitamins,

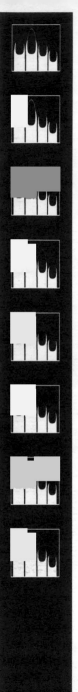

Revlon Salon Professional Nail Builder (which contains calcium), Nail Selectives Rebuild Fortifier or Formula 10 Nail Strengthener.

641. Are strong, healthy nails hereditary?

They can be hereditary, but don't be discouraged if mom doesn't have strong nails. There are many great professional nail products on the market designed to strengthen the nail. Best bets: Nail Selectives Crystal Nail Builder, L'Oreal Salon Professional Mighty Nails and Orly Calcium Shield Nail Builder.

642. Do nail growth products work?

Products applied to the surface of the nail plate do not affect nail growth, because nail growth begins at the matrix of the nail (commonly referred to as the "mother of the nail") deep inside the finger. Massaging cuticle oil or cream into the base of the nail every day will help to stimulate circulation to promote nail growth. Good products to try include: Beauty Secrets Nail Matrix Fortifier, Nail Selectives Rebuild Fortifier, Beauty Secrets Dual Treatment Kit or Contours Botanical Oil.

643. I would like to improve the condition of my nails and hair. Is there a special diet to achieve this?

A good diet can always improve overall health. However, the way to improve the condition of your nails and hair requires more than a good diet. Hair and nails need the right moisturizers or protein. If nails are dry and brittle, they need moisturizing products

like Beauty Secrets Restore Moisturizing Basecoat. If nails are weak and thin, look for products with protein to strengthen the natural nails like Formula 10 Nailteins 2. Also try Nail Nutrition vitamins and supplements for nails. You'll see great results!

644. My nails will grow to a certain length but then begin to chip near the tips. What can I use to strengthen them?

Nails that chip are a result of a number of different things, but usually nails need more nourishment or strength. By using a nail strengthening treatment, nails build up as they grow out. A cuticle conditioner nourishes the nail, since healthy growth begins beneath the cuticle. Good skin care can help, too. Professional skin moisturizing lotions and creams should be part of every basic manicure routine. Natural nail buffers smooth chips and peeling on the nail's free edge to preserve the length until the nail grows out. Nail vitamins can always be used in addition to your manicure routine. Strengthening products include Brucci Miracle Nail Hardener Formaldehyde Free, Windsor Nail Nutrition Tablets and Nail Selectives Rebuild Fortifier.

645. Every time I let my nails grow long they start to crack down the center and split all the way down to the quick. What can I do?

A natural nail capping helps nails grow out and stay strong at the same time. Natural nail cappings can be done with fiberglass, silk, linen or glue and powder applications. Select

a thin and transparent nail capping that is strong, yet looks natural. Try Originails Rap II Fiberglass Nail Wrap Starter Kit or Beauty Secrets Silk Wrap Kit.

646. How can I prevent my nail polish from chipping two or three days after my professional manicure?

Proper home maintenance can ensure longer wearability of a professional manicure. Use products such as cuticle oils or conditioners, professional polishes, topcoats and nail buffers. To prevent chipping, try Brucci Acrylic Shield, Orly Won't Chip Top Coat or Wet Look Glaze.

647. I do not want to have acrylic nails, but do need something to strengthen my nails and keep polish on longer. What is my best option?

Try having them coated with a fiberglass, silk or linen wrap or a powder and glue coating. Called a natural nail capping, this is a thin coating applied to the natural nail only. It strengthens the nail and also helps nail polish stay on the natural nail.

648. What is the best nail color for small hands or someone with long fingers?

All well-manicured natural nails or nail extensions, on small or large hands, can wear any shade that best compliments your skin tone. If you have blue tones in your skin, choose shades with a blue base. If you have yellow tones in your skin, select shades with a yellow/orange base. Do not wear red nail polish on nails that are bitten. If you are uncomfortable with color, sheer shades look very natural.

649. I love bright red polish, but not long nails. Can I wear red on short nails?

Certainly! Pick a shade that compliments your skin tone. For best results, use a professional polish such as Nail Savvy Polish, Nina Polish or Revlon Professional Polish.

650. When is red nail polish not appropriate?

Depending on your lifestyle and the length of your nails, almost all colors are appropriate. Red nail polish is unattractive on bitten nails.

651. What is the difference between a French Manicure and an American Manicure?

In contrast to the stark white tips and "painted" look of French Manicures, the American Manicure Natural Look Polish System gives both nail extensions and natural nails the authentic look of perfectly healthy bare nails wearing only a clear topcoat. Both Orly and Nail Savvy also make products for a French Manicure.

652. I like the look of a French Manicure, but can't always keep my salon appointment. What can I purchase to use at home?

Try American Manicure's French Natural Kit

that contains a guide, two shades of polish, basecoat and topcoat.

653. When polishing my nails, what is the best way to achieve an opaque look with pale polish?

To achieve an opaque look, follow this procedure: First, apply a coat of basecoat, then apply a coat or two of white polish. Apply a single coat of desired color, then finish with topcoat.

654. Which is more drying to my nails, frosted or matte polish?

Since the basic ingredients in frosted and matte polish are the same, neither is more drying to the nails.

655. What is Toluene?

Toluene is an organic solvent that is used in nail polishes, topcoats and basecoats to help the polish stay on the nail. Toluene is included in a list of hazardous chemicals cited in a 1987 California law. A study conducted by the CTFA (Cosmetics, Toiletry and Fragrance Association) produced evidence that the amount of toluene found in nail polish is 10 times below the maximum amount allowed by California law. In other words, the amount of toluene in nail polish does not pose a threat to users. If you are looking for toluene-free nail products, try Revlon's Salon Professional Nail Enamel or Nail Selectives 3/4 ounce Nail Treatments or Nail Savvy Nail Enamel.

656. Why is formaldehyde used in nail products?

Formaldehyde is an ingredient used mostly in nail polish and nail strengtheners to help them dry fast, and acts as a strengthener. Prolonged use of nail products with formaldehyde may cause nails to become brittle, so switch to a non-formaldehyde formula about every 60 days.

657. How many coats of polish are best for a perfect manicure?

For best performance, we recommend one basecoat, two coats of your choice of polish and one topcoat.

658. My polish bubbles up. What causes this?

Several factors can cause nail polish "bubbles." First, be sure to use a professional quality polish. Second, check the age of your polish—old polish will thicken and cause bubbling. Polish thinners are available, but a new bottle is best. Third, never shake your polish bottle because the beads in the bottle can create bubbles. Instead, roll the bottle between your hands. Fourth, if you use a spray-on nail polish dryer, don't hold it too close to the nail or over-spray. Finally, be sure the first coat of polish is completely dry before applying another coat. To thin polish, try Adios Polish Thinner.

659. I have heard that storing nail polish in the refrigerator will prolong the shelf life. Is this true?

No. It is not recommended to store polish in the refrigerator because it can cause it to thicken. Once taken out of the cold, it could take quite awhile to warm up to room temper-

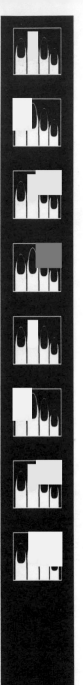

ature. Today's polish formulas and preservatives improve the shelf life of polish. To thin polish that has thickened, add a couple drops of a good nail polish solvent like Gena Professional Nail Polish Thinner.

660. How long does it take to completely dry polish?

How long it takes depends on the type of polish and polish dryer. Generally, it takes one to two hours before nail polish is completely dry. Formaldehyde-free polishes take more time to dry. Many nail polish dryers allow you to use your hands 5 to 15 minutes after polish is applied. However, that doesn't mean heavy gardening!

661. How long should nails dry after a manicure before typing or using a computer?

Today, many nail polish dryers are available that allow you to begin typing or using your computer 5 to 15 minutes after your polish is applied. Topcoat polish drying systems are brushed on over polish color to protect it and speed up drying time. Light-drying systems usually require the use of a specific topcoat and/or basecoat. Do not mix and match different systems, and be sure to follow manufacturer's instructions. Nail drying machines dry polish gently and efficiently with the use of cool or warm air. There are also spray and brush-on polish dryers available. These may be oil-base polish dryers, used on top of the final coat of polish to set it, or oil-free polish dryers, used between coats of polish when it's most important to speed up the drying time. Topcoat polish dryers include Orly's "In a Snap," Nail Selectives Rush Quick Dry/Topcoat and Beauty Secrets Fast Finish

60 Second Polish Dryer/Topcoat. Light-drying systems include Ultra Set. Oil-based dryers include Beauty Secrets Nail Enamel Dryer Spray. Gena's Nail Dry is a non-aerosol, oil-free spray-on dryer.

662. The only time I have to polish my nails is at night before bed. How do I prevent "sheet marks" without losing my sleep?

Today, many nail polish dryers are available that allow you to sleep soundly 5 to 15 minutes after your polish is applied. Included are topcoat polish drying systems, light-drying systems, and spray and brush-on polish dryers. Best bets for sleeping soundly are Varoom Speed Dry, Nail Selective's Rush Super Quick Pro-Dry/Topcoat, Contours Polish Dry and Beauty Secrets Fast Finish 60 Second Polish Dryer/Topcoat.

663. How long must I wait before taking a bath after I've had a manicure?

To prevent smudging, it is best to wait one to two hours before hopping in the tub or shower. A topcoat polish dryer, such as Nail Selectives Rush Super Quick Pro-Dry or Varoom Speed Dry helps nail polish dry faster.

664. How can I get rid of smudges without doing a complete manicure?

Try Claire Topper's Nail Triage which will smooth out little smudges and chips to make your manicure last longer.

665. I want to do something really unusual with my nails. What's a good option to try for special occasions?

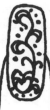

Try Nail Art! Beyond polish, there are a myriad of products for decorating nails. This is called "nail art," some of which, like airbrushing, take a great deal of skill and are best left to the professional. There are a variety of products that make nail art easy for almost anyone. Decals are probably the easiest way to create multicolored designs that look almost like airbrushing. Some come with adhesive backing; others need to be moistened with water. They must be applied to clean, dry nails, which may be previously polished. Foil nail decorations are applied by first coating the nail with a specially formulated glue, sometimes called a foil emulsion. Then the dull side of the foil is pressed onto the nail. When it's lifted away, the colorful side shows. One or more colors of foil can be used together for a "mosaic" effect. Most nail art decoration must be sealed with a special topcoat, often called a bonder or sealer. Follow the manufacturer's instructions exactly for best results. If you want to try nail art yourself, check out Winning Nails 4-Color Airbrush Lace and Foil Decals, Cina Nail Jewelry Decals, Cina Rhinestones, Cina Try Me Nail Art Kit, Eimsuk Fine Art Nail Decals, and Cina Top Coat and Bonder or Winning Nails Tough Coat Bonder/Sealer.

666. I enjoy wearing nail art and want to use a glitter product. How do you apply the glitter so that it stays on the nail?

Purchase a nail art kit containing glitter, like

So Easy Nail Art. To apply the glitter, dip the nail art brush in a clear gloss topcoat, then into the glitter and brush on the nail.

667. Is there a way to remove nail art without removing the polish underneath?

The best way to remove nail art is to also remove the nail polish and start fresh. If you are in a rush, and the nail art is flat on the nail, just apply a coat of polish over the nail art until you have time to remove all of it and start all over.

668. Are decorative nails proper for a wedding, and what type are available?

Nail art can offer a special touch for that special day! Look for festive lace, pearl and gemstone designs, designed with the sophistication appropriate for a day as important as your wedding. Go soft and subtle for your wedding. Remember to follow manufacturer's instructions. For wedding-appropriate designs, try Winning Nails Lace Decals, Foil Decals, and Eimsuk Fine Art Nail Decals for Weddings.

669. What are the pros and cons for having acrylic nails?

Acrylic nails, in most cases, are the strongest semi-permanent nail extensions available. As with all nail extensions, with proper application and proper maintenance there are virtually no negatives to wearing acrylics.

670. What are the benefits of resin coating for nails?

A resin coating with a fabric wrap is a great natural nail strengthener and is better known as nail capping. Resin coating is also generically referred to generically as nail glue, chemically as cyanoacrylate, and technically as adhesive. Most of the time, a resin is used in conjunction with a fabric wrap.

671. Will my acrylic nails yellow like my natural nails when exposed to sunlight?

Generally, nail extensions yellow in the sunlight as a result of the type of basecoat or topcoat used on the nail. The basecoat or topcoat should contain a UV (Ultraviolet) inhibitor to prevent yellowing in the sunlight. Try L'Oreal Salon Professional Top Express or Ultra Set Sunscreen.

672. Will fumes from acrylic nails harm my lungs?

There have never been any recorded cases that state nail product fumes are harmful to the lungs. Remember, anytime a product has a strong odor, even cleaning products in your home, it's recommended these products only be used in well-ventilated areas.

673. How often should my acrylic nails be maintained?

This varies from ten days to three weeks, depending on the growth of your natural nails and how hard you are on the nails.

674. My sculptured nails chip easily at the free edge. Why?

Your sculptured nails may be too long or too thin on the ends for your lifestyle. Have them coated a little thicker or filed a little shorter.

675. My nails won't grow past my finger tips without breaking off. Are nail extensions right for me?

Today, nail extensions can accommodate all lifestyles. Nail extensions are not thick and do not have to be worn long. Today, a more natural look is appealing. There are many different types of extensions such as tips, sculptured nails, nail wraps and gel nails. Consult a professional nail technician to determine which nail extension is best for you.

676. I bought some nail tips and the box said they were "ABS plastic." What does ABS mean?

This is a copolymer of Acrylonitrile-Butadiene-Styrene monomer, from which most artificial nail tips are made.

677. Why do ABS nail tips crack?

Cracking may be due to the wrong style or type selected for your lifestyle, or the tip could be too long. Most nail technicians know a good quality nail tip has "Virgin ABS Plastic" printed on the package. If the package is labeled only "ABS plastic," the tips could be a regrinde, meaning the nail tips will become brittle. Look for Terrific Tips Nail Tips made with Virgin ABS Plastic.

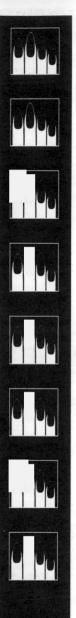

678. I have curved nails and the plastic nail tips I bought won't fit. What should I do?

This style of tip could be the wrong style for the shape of your natural nail. Next time try a tip that has more of a curve like the shape of your own natural nail.

679. Why won't my nail glue stick when I am applying nail tips?

A couple of things may be the cause. If your nail glue is old and stringy, you need to buy a fresh bottle of glue. Also, you may not have applied enough glue to the underside of the tip to have complete coverage under the nail tip.

680. Are tips less harmful to nails than sculptured nails?

Neither one of these types of nail extensions are harmful to the natural nail as long as proper application and proper maintenance procedures are followed. The difference between these two applications is that tips are more temporary, whereas sculptured nails are semi-permanent.

681. I like to wear nail tips. How do I know what size tips to buy to fit my fingers?

When purchasing nail tips, start with an assorted bag. Look at the size number on the tip that fits your nail and write the numbers down so you purchase only the sizes you need. The numbers are encoded, usually 0-9, underneath the tip. The individual refill sizes of Beauty Secrets Oval, Square Form and Exotic Nail Tips are great choices.

682. I am planning a long vacation and want to be prepared to repair or replace a nail tip. What products should I pack?

Take a nail travel kit with you in case you can't get to a salon on your vacation. Pack Beauty Secrets Mini-Tip Kit with tips and glue, add Tropical Shine's 4-Way Buffer, Beauty Secrets Nail Antiseptic, your favorite polish, basecoat and Nail Selectives Rush Quick Dry Top Coat.

683. My nail scissors won't cut my nail tips. What should I use?

It is better to use a toe clipper to trim a tip. Tweezerman's Clean Cut Nail Tip Slicer is made especially for nail tips.

684. Are all nail tips applied in the same way?

No. Application depends on the type of nail tips used. The most common are: full nail tip like OrigiNails Career Length Tips, applied all the way back to the cuticle area; a half-nail tip like Terrific Tips Exotic Lady Extra Overlay Type, applied to half of the natural nail, and usually used with products that are coated over this tip for extra strength; and finally, a nail tip like Electra Nail Jaquar or Contours Extreme Curve Tips, applied to the free edge of the natural nail. This type is also usually used with a coating of product applied over the tip for strength.

685. Can sculptured nails be applied over nail tips?

Yes. This process is commonly referred to as a nail tip with a sculpture or acrylic overlay.

686. Should my manicurist mix and match liquids and powders from different manufacturers to create my sculptured acrylic nails?

NO! Each acrylic system has its own chemical formulation, and the individual components are balanced to work together. If a powder from one manufacturer is used with liquid from another, the nails may take too long to set up, or they may set up too fast and become brittle. Sometimes, combining products that aren't meant to work together can cause uncomfortable heat sensations.

687. I do not want to wear nail extensions any longer. Can I take them off myself?

To properly remove nail extensions, trim the length back to the natural nail length, then file the surface of the nail leaving a thin coating of the product on the nail for strength. This service is best left to a nail technician. Additional oils and moisturizers are used as part of this service to begin strengthening the natural nail to its original state. To help in this transition period, use a good nail strengthener daily, like Beauty Secrets Nail Matrix Fortifier or Contours Botanical Oil.

688. How do I remove my nail tips without tearing my natural nail?

If you are only wearing nail tips that have been applied with nail glue, the simplest way to remove the tips is to trim them back to your natural nail, then use a tip remover like Beauty Secrets Tip and Glue Remover. Apply the tip remover over the seam of the nail tip, allow to set for 3-5 seconds then begin to lift gently. If the nail tip does not lift off, reapply the tip remover. It is important to take your time and do not tear off the nail tip. Follow with a good nail strengthener like Nail Selectives Rebuild Fortifier.

689. I just had my acrylic nails removed and my nails feel as thin as eggshells? What will strengthen them?

If the extensions were removed properly, the eggshell feeling will be temporary. Use a nail strengthener to help toughen them up. Nail and cuticle oils will help plump the layers of the natural nail that have been repeatedly dehydrated by the use of antiseptics in the process of applying extensions. To strengthen nails, try Nail Selectives Rebuild Fortifier or Beauty Secrets Dual Nail Treatment Development System. Contours Botanical Oil helps rehydrate nails. If the nails were removed improperly, the nails won't just feel thin—they will be thin! Every time a nail extension is picked off, pulled off or bitten off, two to three layers of the natural nail plate are forcibly removed. This can actually remove half the thickness of the natural nail! To ensure proper removal of extensions, see your nail professional.

690. Why does my nail technician use a primer?

Nail technicians use a primer to help acrylic nail extension products adhere better to the nail. Primers are special formulations that, if applied improperly, can cause nail damage. Therefore, it is a good idea to leave the application of primers in the hands of the nail technicians. Not all nail extensions require

the use of a primer. Wrapped nails, such as fiberglass, silk and linen, or glue and powder applications do not require the application of a primer.

691. Why does the primer burn sometimes, and how can it be stopped?

Sometimes primer may cause a burning sensation if too much is applied to nails which have recently been in strong cleaning solutions, have had nail extensions removed incorrectly, or have very thin, sensitive nail beds. First, determine if the actual nail bed is burning or if it is the cuticle area around the nail. It is important to understand that the burning is caused because most primers contain acid. If the nail bed is burning, the nail technician may apply an antiseptic to the nail and may consider discontinuing the use of primer during future nail services. If the cuticle area is burning, then it may be neutralized with an over-the-counter antacid product. Remember, primer should be used VERY SPARINGLY. It is very easy to apply too much and have it run onto the surrounding cuticle area.

692. Why do my nail beds hurt and my cuticles look red and puffy after I have nail extensions applied?

This can be caused by excessive filing. The file used on your nails also may have been too coarse. Be sure to tell your nail technician you have sensitive nails. Red puffy cuticles may also be caused by a reaction to products used on your nails. Consult your nail technician to prevent problems like this.

693. I wear extensions, but they keep lifting up. What's wrong?

Lifting is caused by several things, such as nails shaped with deep indentations or unusually high arches; not using an antiseptic to clean, sanitize and dehydrate the natural nail before applying the nail extension; using products with mineral oil and lanolin on hands; not pushing back the cuticle properly when applying extensions; or taking certain prescription medications. Hormonal changes in the body (such as menopause), as well as excessive stress can also contribute to lifting. When applying nail tips, be sure to select the correct size, and use a good nail glue. If the glue looks stringy, it is too old and won't work properly. On acrylic nails, be sure to use non-acetone polish removers because acetone may cause them to lift. Acrylic nails are best applied by a professional nail technician.

694. My acrylic nails look like cracked ice. What happened?

If this happens during the application of the product, it is due to the cold temperature of the product, the room in which you are working or the temperature of the hands. If the product has been stored in a cold area, it must be warmed to room temperature before using. If the hands are cold, warm them before starting the procedure. If the room is cold, adjust the temperature or work directly under a lamp. If the cracking occurs after application, it may be due to old product.

695. My acrylic nails have started to yellow. What causes this?

Many acrylics change color to a yellow cast just from wearing them for a long period of time or if a basecoat is not being used under polish. Look for the new acrylic products with UV (ultraviolet) inhibitors that help prevent acrylic nails from turning dingy yellow. Check out Ultra Set's Sun Screen for Nails or L'Oreal Salon Professional Top Coat Express.

696. If I wear nail extensions for a long period of time will my nails be ruined?

Wearing nail extensions won't ruin your natural nails. The improper application, maintenance, and most important, the improper removal of nail extensions can damage natural nails.

697. What's the difference between a linen, silk or fiberglass wrap? Is one better or stronger than the other?

Linen provides excellent strength but is not very thin or transparent. Silk looks the most natural and offers flexibility, but may be too delicate for people who are hard on their hands. Fiberglass provides the best of both worlds with the natural look of silk, plus the strength of linen. Silk and fiberglass often come with an adhesive backing, available in sheets, strips and pre-cut fingers. Try Beauty Secrets Silk or Fiberglass Nail Wrap Kits or Gena Brush-On Fiberglass Wrap System.

698. What is the difference between a liquid nail wrap and a silk or linen nail wrap?

A liquid wrap contains tiny fibers of a fabric, like nylon. It's a little like a "nail wrap in a bottle." It coats nails to give them extra thickness to reinforce them. Liquid wraps are great for easy maintenance and quick repairs on natural nails. Try Super Nail Liquid Wrap or Orly's Romeo Instant Nail Wrap. A fabric nail wrap is a semi-permanent nail extension. A thin layer of fabric is cut to size and glued onto the nail to add strength, and sometimes length.

699. What is nail wrapping?

A nail wrap is a semi-permanent nail extension that is a thin layer of silk, linen or fiberglass or fabric, cut to size and glued onto the nail to add strength, and sometimes length. Wraps can be done on natural nails or as a tip overlay, which is the most common. Usually, one layer of fabric is applied and then one or more layers of glue are applied on top to provide strength.

700. My nails are constantly splitting. Is there a product that can protect my nails?

Nail care products containing nylon fibers, when applied to the natural nail, can provide external thickening and temporary strengthening. Since the added strength is temporary, it is recommended these products be applied with every manicure to provide consistent strength as your nails grow longer. Try SuperNail Fiber Nail Wrap with Fibers or Nail Selectives Silk Fill.

701. I'm worried about getting an infection from a manicure. What should my manicurist do to prevent the spread of infection?

The best insurance against infection is for your manicurist to previously sanitize each implement used during your manicure, and to cleanse and dehydrate your natural nails as extra security. If you think you have a fungal infection, tell your manicurist. She should not apply nail extension products.

702. There are so many different nail glue products, how do I know which one to use?

Most nail glues have a thin viscosity designed for applying nail tips or mending nails. Try Beauty Secrets Quick Dry or Super Nail Stick It nail glue. Thicker glues are used for wraps because they take longer to dry so the wrap can be positioned properly. A nail glue accelerator like OrigiNails Rap Dry speeds up drying. Try 5-Second Wrap Glue or Beauty Secrets Wrap Set Glue if wrapping nails.

703. What is the best product for sanitizing manicure utensils?

Isopropyl alcohol will sanitize your personal implements. Regulations for disinfecting implements used in a salon vary by state. Most states require use of a hospital-grade disinfectant, such as Barbicide Plus.

704. Can the AIDS virus be transmitted during a manicure?

The AIDS virus is transmitted only by the exchange of bodily fluids. There is a remote possibility that the virus could be transmitted if an AIDS-contaminated nipper or other instrument draws blood on a client. Proper sterilization of implements prevents this.

705. How do I know my manicurist is sanitizing her manicure utensils properly before using them on me?

Sanitation in the salon is a big issue today. Ask your nail technician to show you how he or she sanitizes their implements. The implements should be submerged in a sanitizing solution like Barbicide and never used on more than one client before being sanitized. If you are still uncertain about proper sanitation, purchase your own set of professional nail implements and take them with you to every salon visit. A good choice is the Protech Professional Tool Kit with cuticle nippers, scissors, nail clippers, cuticle pusher and emery file.

706. What is a "light-drying" system?

This could refer to gel nails that can only be cured or dried under an ultraviolet light, or one of the new topcoat drying systems, like Ultra Set. This is a quick-dry topcoat applied to nails, then cured or dried by placing nails under a hand-held ultraviolet light. This system creates a harder, glossier finish than most air-dried topcoats.

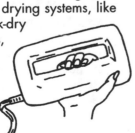

707. What should I do if nail glue gets on my skin?

It is always a good idea to have a glue remover on hand, like Super Nail Glue Off or Beauty Secrets Tip and Glue Remover. If you're in a pinch, you can use acetone, polish remover or run hot water where skin has glue. If your fingers are glued together, never pull them apart.

708. How does my manicurist get the nail glue to dry so quickly when she is doing wraps on my nails?

Your nail technician is using a product called a "glue accelerator" or "activator." This product instantly dries nail glue during wrap or powder and glue applications.

709. Instead of having my nails wrapped, is it true that I can just apply nail glue to my natural nails to strengthen them?

Yes. Nail glue is the thinnest application of a natural nail strengthener that can be used. Easy brush-on glues include Beauty Secrets No-Mix Brush-On Glaze or the Rap II Brush-on Glue. For quick applications, use Beauty Secrets No-Mix Brush-On Dry or Rap II Brush-On Accelerator to dry the Brush-On Glue.

710. I love my gel nails. They never break or lift. What is the difference between gels and acrylics?

Gels and acrylics are chemically different, and are applied differently to nails. The application you choose should be determined by

your nail type, lifestyle and activities. However, one type of product or application is not necessarily better than the other.

711. Can I use regular nail glue to fill in my gel extensions?

Nail glues and no-light gels are chemically similar, in that they are both cyanoacrylates, but they have different viscosities. Therefore, it won't do any damage to interchange them. For best results, always repair and fill gel extensions with the same gel used to create them. To fill gel extensions, try Gena Brush-On Nail Gel System, Gena Brush-On No-Light Nail Gel or Super Nail No-Lite Gel. Gel extensions applied using an ultraviolet light contain a different chemical, so you should not use regular nail glue on them.

712. Will nail gels burn my nails when they are being "cured" under a light?

Most likely this will not happen unless you have very sensitive nail beds. If this does happen, take your hands out from under the light, wait a few minutes, then put your hands back under the light. This should eliminate the sensitivity.

713. I just had my manicurist apply gel nails and within a few days they started to lift. What causes this and how can lifting be prevented?

There are many things that can cause lifting. Consult with your nail technician and have the nails reapplied. Be certain to keep in mind that simple things like mineral oil, suntan oils and some cleaning solutions can cause lifting to all nail extensions.

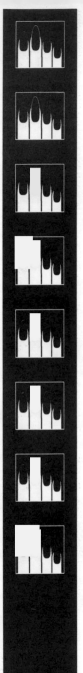

714. When my manicurist applied gels to my nails I felt like they were on fire! What causes this, and do I need to give up wearing gel nails?

No, you don't need to give up wearing nail extensions. Gel nails may not be the right type of nails for you. The "burning sensation" or a heat sensation that you felt under the light is what is called photosensitivity. If this happens again, just take your hand out from under the light, wait a few minutes, then put your hand back under the light. You will find the burning sensation is gone. There are also gel systems that are called "No Light" gels. These systems use a thicker viscosity glue and cure or "dry" the glue with an accelerator.

715. My gel nail lifted once and exposed my natural nail. My natural nail is still very strong. Why do acrylics make nails so weak and gels keep nails at their natural strength?

Acrylic nails will not damage your natural nails if they are applied and maintained properly. One difference between acrylics and gels is that most acrylics require the use of a primer and most gels do not. If a primer is improperly used, nails could become weak.

716. My hands are in the water a lot. I am afraid all the moisture might cause a nail fungus. What should I do?

Being in water should not cause nail fungus. Nail fungus can be prevented with proper application and maintenance of nail exten-

sions. If a nail extension has lifted and you need a quick fix, be certain not to just glue the nail, especially if your hands have been in water. First, use a blow dryer to completely dry under the nail. Then apply a nail antiseptic like OrigiNails Steri Nail to the exposed area of the nail, which will help prevent nail problems. Finish by applying nail glue under the lifted area of the nail extension, like Beauty Secrets Nail Glue Plus with a special moisture-reducing agent.

717. How can a nail fungus be detected?

You cannot detect a nail fungus before it happens. However you can help prevent one from happening. If a nail fungus occurs, it will appear to be a white area under the nail, as if the natural nail is pulling away from the nail bed. Proper application and maintenance of the nail extensions and using products like a nail antiseptic will help prevent a nail fungus.

718. How can nail mold be detected?

You cannot detect a nail mold before it happens. However, you can help prevent one from occurring. If a nail mold occurs, it appears as a brownish or greenish-color on the natural nail. It is caused by moisture being trapped between an extension and the natural nail due to lifting. Proper application and maintenance of nail extensions and using a nail antiseptic, like Beauty Secrets Nail Antiseptic, No Lift Nails Fung Off or SuperNail Protect Anti-Infection Nail Oil, can help prevent nail mold.

719. How do I get rid of that green mold on my nail?

Consult with your nail technician. She will probably remove the nail extension and file the surface of the nail. Your nail technician will not be able to completely file the discoloration off of the nail. It will need to grow off. Once the nail has been filed, it is treated with a nail antiseptic. Depending on the severity, product may be reapplied.

720. What is the best way to get rid of a nail fungus?

The best way to treat a nail fungus is to consult with your nail technician. They will probably advise you to see your physician.

721. Is a nail fungus contagious?

A nail fungus may be contagious. If it is not taken care of properly, it could spread to other fingers. If an implement or nail file is used on a nail with a fungus and then used on another person, the fungus could also be spread.

722. What is the best antiseptic for use for your manicure tools?

There are several implement sanitizing products on the market, such as Wahl Clini-Clip Clipper Blade Disinfectant, Oster Spray Disinfectant and Barbicide. Be certain to read the package and follow the manufacturer's instructions carefully.

723. What is the difference between acetone and non-acetone nail polish remover? Which is best?

Acetone polish removers are for use on natural nails. Non-acetone polish removers contain ethyl acetate or nethyl ethyl keytone as their active ingredient and were developed for use with nail extensions because acetone can cause extensions to become brittle and "lift."

724. Will I damage my nails if I peel off my nail polish instead of using nail polish remover?

Any time you are picking or peeling anything from the surface of the nail, you may not see an immediate difference, but it will eventually cause a problem by making the natural nail thinner. If you are looking for easy ways to remove polish, try Gena Zip Off Nail Polish Remover.

725. How can a pedicure keep my feet healthy?

Regular pedicures help keep feet looking pretty and prevent dry skin and calluses. Start with a 10 minute soak using a foot bath or soak. Dry skin sloughing lotions and special foot files remove dry skin and calluses. Pedicure lotions, powders and cooling gels (a refreshing treatment) pamper the feet. In addition, special antiseptic, antifungal foot sprays are available if treatment for fungus is necessary. A coarse grit file can be useful for tough toenails. And a professional quality polish is the finishing touch for any good pedicure. Perfect Feet offers a complete line of professional pedicure products.

726. I have calluses and thickened skin on my heels. How can I get rid of this unsightly problem?

Treat yourself to a regular pedicure. Use a sloughing lotion or special foot file to remove dry skin and calluses. Using these regularly will begin to eliminate those calluses. Also, using a pumice stone can greatly reduce unsightly calluses and dry patches. Try Gena's "Perfect Feet Pedicure" System, Winning Nails Fancy Foot Pedicure File and Tweezerman Pedicure Callus Shaver for extra thick skin and calluses, which safely shaves away dry, dead skin. Follow manufacturer's directions carefully.

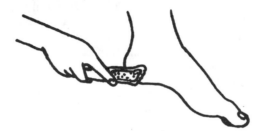

727. How should my toenails be trimmed? Straight or rounded?

Toenails should be trimmed and filed straight and never too short. This will help to prevent ingrown toenails.

728. What is the best tool for clipping my toenails?

Professional heavy-duty stainless steel toenail clippers by Revlon or Tweezerman should be used because of the thickness of the toenail.

729. Can fingernails and toenails get sunburned?

No. Natural nails and toenails do not get sunburned. Polished nails that are not coated with a topcoat that contains a UV inhibitor can turn yellow and discolor the polish. UV-inhibiting topcoats include Beauty Secrets Fast Finish and Beauty Secrets Nail Hardener and Thickener.

730. My toenails turn yellow. What should I do to whiten them?

Yellow and stained toenails can be caused by wearing polish without a basecoat, or your nails may appear yellow if you've worn clear or sheer polishes without a UV inhibitor in the sun. A consultation with your nail professional can help determine the cause. Use Gena's Nail Brite Whitening Scrub, which contains a mild abrasive, or Varoom Lemon Brite Cuticle Remover, which contains an ingredient like lemon juice to easily eliminate discoloration.

731. How can I prevent my pale nail polish from turning yellow in the sun?

Use a polish topcoat that contains an ultra-violet inhibitor to prevent pale polishes from changing colors or turning yellow, check out Beauty Secrets Nail Hardener and Thickener, Beauty Secrets Fast Finish Dryer Topcoat and Nail Selectives Crystal Nail Builder.

732. Will my nails turn yellow if I wear polish for a long period of time?

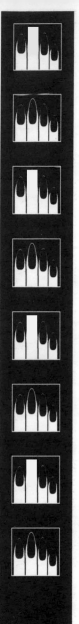

It can happen. Prevent this common situation by applying a basecoat before applying nail polish to nails.

733. When I remove my red nail polish, my nails seem to stay pink for weeks. Is there a product available that will take the stain off?

The pink discoloration on the natural nail is due to the pigmentation of the red polish. To help prevent discoloration, use a professional basecoat. To remove the stain from the natural nail, use Gena's Nail Brite. Stain-preventing basecoats include Nail Selectives Hydra-Coat Base Coat and Orly Top 2 Bottom. Try Ultra Set's Natural Nail Adhesive, a water-based basecoat that not only prevents staining, but also works on natural nails to actually keep polish on longer.

734. What causes my natural nails to discolor after I wear certain colors of nail polish like reds and burgundies?

This is not a reaction to the polish. To prevent this, use a basecoat before applying polish. If you already have a problem with discolored natural nails, try Gena Nail Brite to help remove the discoloration. Try Nail Selectives Hydra Coat Basecoat or European Secrets Stix Molecular Basecoat.

735. I am a lifeguard and am consequently in the sun a lot. What can I do to keep my nails from yellowing?

There are polish topcoats available that contain an ultraviolet inhibitor to help prevent

natural nails from yellowing. Also, these topcoats help prevent lighter polishes from changing colors or turning yellow. Try Beauty Secrets Fast Finish or Beauty Secrets Nail Hardener and Thickener.

736. I have stopped and started smoking numerous times in the past 20 years. Each time I start and stop smoking again, I notice that my nails yellow. Is this possible, and what can I do to correct it?

Yellow and stained nails can be caused by smoking or by wearing polish without a basecoat. Your nails may appear yellow if you've worn clear or sheer polishes without a UV inhibitor in the sun. A consultation with your nail professional can help determine the cause. A thorough buffing with a fine grit nail file may be enough to remove the yellow. If not, use a nail scrub which contains a mild abrasive or use Gena's Nail Brite Whitening Scrub, which contains an ingredient, like lemon juice, to easily eliminate discoloration.

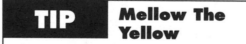

Mellow The Yellow

For yellowing nails or tips, wrap cotton around the end of a cuticle pusher and moisten with hydrogen peroxide. Run along the underside of nail to whiten and brighten!

737. What's the quickest and best way to fix a broken nail?

There are many quick-mending products available for natural nails, such as nail glues. If the natural nail is split, mend it with a tempo-

rary-fix, like Beauty Secrets Nail Glue. If the natural nail is broken, look for products that will extend the length of the nail as a temporary fix. If you are wearing nail extensions and one broke, look for "emergency repair" kits. It is always best to have your professional nail technician repair and maintain your nails. For emergencies, keep on hand Beauty Secrets Nail Glue, plus Beauty Secrets Wrap Kits in Silk or Fiberglass, 5-Second Nail Repair Kit or the Nails-To-Go Travel Repair Kit.

738. What is a pumice stone?

Pumice is a light, porous stone, formed by the escape of steam from cooling volcanic lava. Pumice stones can be used to remove rough, dry, built-up patches or calluses after the skin has been soaked in warm water to pre-soften. Try Flowery Pumice Stone or Moom's Black Natural Pumice Stone.

739. My manicurist warms a lotion before I soak my hands in it. Can I do the same at home to moisturize my hands and nails?

Yes. Moisturizing hands should be a part of home maintenance. Consider purchasing a manicuring hot oil machine such as Gena's Warm-O-Lator and Gena's Adios Warm-O-Lotion. Be certain to follow manufacturer's directions. Tip: Rub Adios Warm-O-Lotion on hands before going to sleep at night. Cover hands with white cotton Beauty Gloves. Hands soften while you sleep!

740. What is a paraffin wrap?

Paraffin is a waxy substance used in heat

treatments by manicurists and aestheticians. Warm paraffin is used to coat the hands, feet or face. This paraffin coating holds heat in for 10 to 15 minutes and causes the pores to open to allow moisturizers to penetrate into the skin more readily. Paraffin therapy conditions and softens the cuticles and leaves hands feeling soft and pampered.

741. Does a moisturizer help keep nails healthy?

Moisture loss is a major cause of nail brittleness and breakage. A daily moisturizing treatment for hands and nails keeps moisture loss to a minimum. The more your hands and nails are exposed to drying elements (like dish washing, the sun or handling paperwork) the more frequently you should moisturize. Look for cuticle oils and creams designed specifically to moisturize the cuticle. Using these products regularly also stimulates blood circulation in the matrix which helps to promote healthy nail growth. Try these moisturizing products: Contours Botanical Oil or Gena's Healthy Hoof Nail Treatment.

742. I use hand lotion but my hands continue to get very rough and red. What is a good treatment for this kind of problem?

Hands tend to get more rough and red in the winter because your hands are drier than at any other time of the year. The massaging action stimulates blood circulation throughout the hands and arms and promotes the absorption of conditioners into the skin. Be certain to apply hand creams frequently, more than once a day if your hands are very dry. Always apply creams after washing your hands or submerging them in water. Try Triple Lanolin's Hand and Nail Conditioner, Purist Swedish Herbal Hand Cream or Aromesentials Vitamin E and Alderflower Hand and Body Lotion. New products are the hand lotions containing alpha hydroxy acids which are designed to speed exfoliation of dead skin cells, like Purist Skin Therapy Hand and Body Lotion.

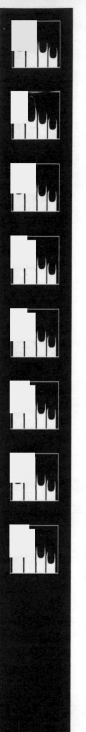

Beauty Diary

NAIL IT

CHAPTER TEN

Hair Raising Answers

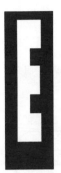

Ever since the days of the caveman, some form of sharp implement has been used to remove hair. From primitive sharpened flints to collections of prized bronze razors, hair removal tools have been regarded as essential to good grooming.

Modern technology has made the often painful task of hair removal easier, and in many cases, much less painful, thanks to the invention of the safety razor in 1762. For centuries, women endured nicks, scrapes and burns when having their unwanted body hair plucked, waxed, pulled and scraped off. And although in the early 20th century women could borrow from the boys those Schick, Gillette or Sunbeam razors, it wasn't until 1940 that Remington rolled out the first electric shaver specifically designed for women.

Today, in most modern societies, smooth, shiny skin is not only a sign of good health, but also good grooming.

Women tweeze their eyebrows to suit the latest fashion trend. They shave, wax and depilate hair on legs, under arms, above the lip and in the delicate "bikini" area. All in the name of "beauty."

743. What method do dermatologists recommend for removing unwanted hair?

Electrolysis is suggested for sparse, unwanted hair. For more abundant hair, waxing is best. Seek a recommendation for a good electrologist from your dermatologist.

744. I have heavy, dark hair on my arms. Should I bleach or remove the hair?

This is usually a matter of personal preference. If you choose bleaching, Invisi-Bleach is specially formulated for this purpose.

745. What is the best way to remove hair using a hand-held electrolysis machine?

Hair should be 1/6 to 1/2 inch long. Take a hot shower or hot bath to soften hairs. Pull skin taut while depilling hair. Consider waxing hair first, then using the machine for keeping the area hair-free as hair grows in.

746. What is the difference between the paraffin used to soften hands and the wax used for hair removal?

Paraffin wax is lanolin-enriched and contains moisturizing oils. Gigi Honee Wax is made with clover honey and other natural resins which facilitate hair removal.

747. Why does it hurt when I get my legs waxed? Can the pain be lessened?

Leg hair is pulled off with the wax. To help ease the pain, skin should be pulled very taut in the opposite direction the wax strip will be removed. Stretching the skin properly is the most important tip for reducing pain. Be sure to use a pre-conditioning lotion like GiGi Pre-Hon Pre-Epilation Lotion with special anti-inflammatory agents that protect sensitive skin from irritation. Immediately after the wax is removed, apply firm pressure to the area with your hands. The sting can also be lessened at the point by placing an ice-cold pack where hair was removed.

748. I don't take time to use shaving cream when I shave my legs. What else could I use that would be faster and more conditioning to my legs?

Surgi-Cream makes a gel called Smooth Shave that is formulated especially for women. It contains aloe vera, Vitamin E and collagen to condition while you shave. You could also use a body oil like Freeman's Aromesenstials Hazelnut & Sesame prior to shaving.

749. How long should my hair be to be waxed?

Hair should be 1/2 inch long the first time for the wax to take hold.

750. How do you get unmelted wax out of the well of the waxing machine?

Use Gigi Sure Clean All Purpose Cleaner and a soft cloth.

751. What hair removal technique lasts the longest?

Waxing lasts longer than other methods, especially when a warm wax is used, because it penetrates into the pores and pulls out the entire hair from the root. On the average, it takes three to six weeks for the hair to grow back. For permanent hair removal, electrolysis is recommended.

752. Can I wax my legs at home effectively?

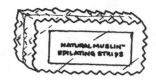

You can wax your legs at home, but probably not as effectively as a professional can. Hot wax kits for home use can be messy. However, Gigi Microwave Kit is an efficient system providing a transparent wax so that you can see exactly which hairs have been covered by the wax. Care should be taken in heating the wax, and be sure to closely follow the manufacturer's instructions. The Clean & Easy Mini Waxer is easy to use because the wax is applied with a roll-on applicator that eliminates mess. Hair is removed with cloth strips almost as effectively as in a professional waxing salon. You might also want to try the cold wax strips, like Clean & Easy Strip Wax or Gigi Hair Removal Strip, in which wax is spread on strips that you press on and pull off. The downside: cold wax sometimes does not strip all the hair off.

753. What is safer, waxing or bleaching?

If done according to manufacturers' directions, both are safe.

754. Can I get skin damage from waxing with the wax too hot?

If directions are followed correctly, you won't damage your skin. Always test hot wax on the inside of your arm for warmth prior to applying to a large area. Also, when using a new product, always do a patch test for possible skin allergies.

755. I waxed my legs, but all the hair did not come off. What happened?

This could be a result of several things. the wax was not hot enough; the hairs were too short to imbed in the wax; the angle at which the strip was pulled was wrong—it should have been at a 40° angle; or the strip was not pulled off quickly enough. Hair must be at least 1/2 inch long for waxing.

756. What causes redness, swelling or skin irritation after waxing?

The cause could be that the wax was not warm enough, the wax remover was pulled straight up and not parallel to the skin, the skin was not held taut when pulling off the strip, the waxing was done too soon after bathing or showering, or deodorants were used after waxing. Wait 12 hours to use deodorant.

757. How long will my skin stay smooth after using a depilatory?

That depends on your hair type, whether you have strong, coarse or fine hair. Skin will stay smooth usually two to six weeks because depilatories reach hair just below the surface.

758. How do I remove an ingrown hair or splinter without damaging my skin?

Use a sharply pointed tweezer like Tweezerman's Ingrown Hair Remover. Use the point to spring out the hair, then tweeze. Clean the area with hydrogen peroxide. Wait at least 15 minutes before applying creams or moisturizers.

759. How long after waxing should I wait before going out in the sun?

Twenty-four hours is recommended unless you use sunscreen.

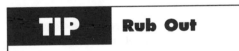

TIP | **Rub Out**

To prevent ingrown hairs between shaving or waxing, rub shaved areas vigorously with a towel every time you bathe.

760. Will salt water irritate my skin if I have had my legs waxed?

Wait 24 hours to take the plunge to avoid irritation.

761. Why do depilatory creams smell so bad?

Depilatory creams contain two powerful chemical compounds, sodium thioglycolate and calcium thioglycolate, which both can dissolve keratin—what hair is made of.

Sometimes the smell is worse after the depilatory is applied because the thioglycolate acid reacts with the hair to create a sulphur-type by-product—the bad egg smell! A few formulations are available which are not as strong smelling, such as Clean & Easy Cream Depilatory.

762. What do I do if my skin breaks out after using a depilatory?

Wash with Betadine and follow with Neosporin cream or a cortisone spray to reduce inflammation. Betadine is an antibacterial cleanser that is available over-the-counter from your pharmacist.

763. Will depilatories dry my skin?

Depilatories are not drying if you follow up with a finishing cream or balm, such as Palm Beach Skin Saver with aloe vera to soothe and moisturize skin.

764. When should I shave? Morning or the night before?

Shave at night to reduce redness.

765. When should I shave my legs before going to the beach?

Wait 12 hours after shaving or waxing to plunge into the spa, pool, lake or ocean. Shaving stubble is the one drawback of shaving, although it is still the most popular method for removing leg and bikini hair.

766. What is the proper way to shave my legs?

When shaving or using a wax, hair should always be removed in the opposite direction hair grows.

767. How can I prevent the redness and stinging that occurs after I shave my legs?

Wash your razor and legs with Betadine before shaving. Shave in the shower using Surgi-Clean Shave Gel which softens the hairs to make shaving easier. After shaving, use Gigi Antiseptic Lotion to moisturize the skin. Palm Beach Skin Saver helps minimize redness and irritation, and leaves skin feeling smooth and cool because it is enriched with aloe vera.

768. Can I easily remove hair from the "bikini" area?

Shaving may be the easiest, but it is not the most effective way to remove bikini-area hair. The best way is to have hair professionally removed using a waxing product. If this is not possible, try Clean & Easy Bikini Roll On or Clean & Easy Wax Strips, which can be used at home.

769. What is the best way to remove facial hair myself?

Ardell Surgi-Cream and Clean & Easy Brush-On Facial Hair Remover dissolve the hair at the skin level. Another easy-to-use solution is Gigi Hair Removal Strips for the face.

770. I noticed a slight darkening of hair on my upper lip. What causes this, and how can I get rid of it without shaving?

It is caused by hormonal changes in your body which can happen anytime in a woman's life, but especially after menopause. Try a gentle depilatory like Surgi-Cream, or facial wax like Clean & Easy Facial Strip Wax or bleaching with a facial bleach like Invisi-Bleach.

771. If I trim my facial hair, will it grow back thicker?

No. Trimming only cuts the hair shaft. It does not affect the way it grows.

772. How can I prevent those tiny red bumps in the bikini area after shaving?

Use a moisturizing product like Surgi-Cream Gel while shaving, follow with Gigi Antiseptic Lotion to refine pores and Gigi Benzokal Lotion with allantoin to calm skin.

773. What is the best method to remove or minimize those unsightly hairs that grow in the nose and ears?

Nose hair should be clipped with tiny manicure scissors or Tweezerman's blunt nose scissors made especially for this task. For easier hair removal, Wahl makes a battery-operated nose hair trimmer. Nose hairs should not be waxed! Ear hairs can be waxed or tweezed, but it is quite uncomfortable. Most good stylists usually will clip the ear hairs when they are trimming the hair. At home, have your spouse, roommate or significant other tweeze or trim the hairs for you, since it is hard to do it yourself.

774. How do I choose tweezers, especially when there are so many shapes?

For long-lasting tweezers, choose a professional quality, 100 percent stainless steel tweezer that will not rust when cleaned. The prongs should have a light, gentle spring action and the gripping platforms (at the tips) should be smooth and polished. When the tips are pressed together, they should meet perfectly. Tweezerman makes a variety. Selecting the shape is a matter of personal preference.

775. What is the most ideal tweezer to use to tweeze my brows?

Tweezerman's slant point tweezer is the most popular tweezer to use, although there are square and fine point varieties which are ideal for tweezing very fine hairs.

776. How can I reduce the irritation from having my brows tweezed?

Dampen a cotton ball with a mild astringent, like Sea Breeze, and gently wipe the area to be tweezed to help prevent infection. Take a steamy shower or place a hot washcloth over your brow before tweezing to open the pores. Don't use an ice cube or "freeze before you tweeze," because this will close the pores and it makes it harder to pull the hair. Use a moisturizer after, not before tweezing, so you are sure to get a good grip on the hair.

777. If you numb the skin in the eyebrow area, will this eliminate pain when arching the eyebrows?

Numbing (with ice) closes the pores, making it harder to pull the hair—hence more pain. Taking a steamy shower or placing a hot washcloth over your brows prior to tweezing opens the pores to make tweezing much more comfortable.

778. Is it true that overplucked eyebrows won't grow back?

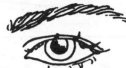

No. The only way to keep hair from growing back is to destroy the hair root (papilla), which is usually done by electrolysis. It can take plucked hairs up to eight weeks to grow back.

779. What is the best way to tweeze my brows?

First, brush the hairs in the direction of the hair growth. Isolate the hair you want to tweeze. Always tweeze in the direction of the hair growth. Pull ONE hair at a time, gently and smoothly. Do not yank the hair out. Ouch! Brows should start just above the inner corner of the eye and extend slightly past the outer corner of the eye.

TIP **Quick Shave**

For a smooth, quick, dry-shave clean-up on legs, rub Clubman Shave Cream on areas you wish to shave. When finished shaving, wipe off excess cream with towel or washcloth. Legs feel fresh and smooth, thanks to the aloe vera in the cream.

Beauty Diary

HAIR RAISING ANSWERS

CHAPTER ELEVEN

Sensational Skin

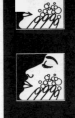

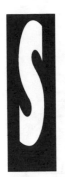

Since ancient times, bathing and care of the skin have enjoyed a history of elaborate ritual, going far beyond basic health and hygiene. The Egyptians, Romans and Greeks elevated bathing to a luxurious art, one that is still enjoyed today!

In Egypt, it was common for women to take a series of daily baths from cold to hot, followed by an aromatic, oil-infused facial and body massages. Skin softening oils were scented with frankincense, myrrh, thyme, marjoram and fruit or nut essences. In fact, clay tablets dating back to 3000 B.C. reveal such beauty recipes as a mixture of bullock's bile, whipped ostrich eggs, olive oil, flour, sea salt, plant resin and fresh milk as an antidote for blemishes. Wrinkle relief came in the form of a paste of milk, incense, wax, olive oil, gazelle or crocodile dung and ground juniper leaves.

Although Greek women adopted much of the Egyptian toilette, it was the Romans who established bathing as an important social ritual. Around the 2nd century B.C., Romans built enormous bathing complexes for men, including gardens, exercise rooms, shops, libraries and lounges, not unlike today's more elaborate spas and health clubs. Although similar but smaller facilities were available to women, Roman ladies were usually attended to at home by slaves known as "cosmetae." After bathing, the face was massaged and painted. Finally, the neck and shoulders were rubbed with scented oils and the body washed in rose water.

The invention of cold cream can be attributed to the Greek physician Galen in the 2nd century. His formula called for one part white wax melted into three parts olive oil, in which "rose buds had been steeped and as much water as can be blended into the mass." Galen recommended lanolin as an alternative, derived from sheep's wool, an ingredient still widely used as a skin softener today.

While bathing was commonplace throughout the Roman Empire, northern Europeans were never as enthusiastic about bathing. It was believed to be a health hazard due to the colder climate, and considered evil to expose the flesh. Such poor hygiene contributed to widespread disease throughout Europe. It was not until the 19th century when bathing was understood as important to the prevention of disease that bathing become a common practice.

Today, we combine bathing and skin care rituals—even some of the ingredients—used by ancient civilizations with the scientific know-how of modern technology. Scientists have even come to understand how and why ancient beauty preparations were effective. We know now that when Egyptians took milk baths and Romans bathed in aged wine, they were having an alpha hydroxy acid treatment!

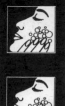

780. My skin is dry. Should I use a rinseable or a cream-based cleanser? How often?

Dry skin can be cleaned twice daily with a non-soap cleansing bar, a rinseable lotion formulated for dry skin or a cleansing cream. Toilet soap tends to be drying, so it is not recommended. For a rinseable cleanser, try Purist Citrus Aloe Rinse Off Cleansing Milk or Milk'N Honee Facial Wash for All Skin Types. Work up a lather using very gentle circular motions with your finger tips. Rinse thoroughly to hydrate your skin and remove all traces of cleanser. Apply a moisturizer immediately. Cleansing creams are particularly good for thoroughly removing makeup. Try Purist Fresh Lemon Deep Pore Cleansing Cream or Purist Skin Therapy Perfecting Cleanser. If your skin is very dry and sensitive, the wood fibers in the tissues used to remove cleansing cream may irritate your skin. If so, try wiping your cleansing cream off with a soft, lukewarm cloth. If you have very dry skin, try using a cleansing cream at night and a rinseable cleanser in the morning. Pat dry with a towel and apply a moisturizer such as Purist Skin Therapy Day Moisture Cream immediately to lock in moisture.

781. What is the most effective way to clean normal skin?

For normal skin, avoid extremes—products that are either drying or oily. Wash your face in the morning and before bed with either a soap-based or a non-soap cleanser, such as Freeman Professional's Aromesentials Lime Blossom and Yogurt Cleansing Milk for normal skin. Using gentle, circular motions, work up a lather with your finger tips or a soft cloth. Rinse thoroughly, pat dry and apply a light moisturizer, such as Freeman Professional's Aromesentials Butter Rose and Chamomile Moisturizer.

782. I have oily skin, how can I best cleanse it?

For oily skin, cleanse two to three times daily using a bar or lotion cleanser formulated for oily skin. (Avoid oil-based cleansing creams.) Try Jheri Redding Milk'N Honee Beauty Bar or Aromesentials Ginger and Comfrey Gel Cleanser or Aromesentials Alpha Hydroxy bar soap. Use a soft cloth or your finger tips to work up a lather. Rinse thoroughly to remove all traces of product and towel dry. Following cleansing, moisten a quilted cotton pad with a toner or astringent, such as Purist Clarifying Skin Toner. Wipe pad across oily areas of face. If skin is very oily, use a toner or astringent as needed during the day to control excess oil.

783. I have combination skin. What is the best way to cleanse it?

If you have combination skin, your skin is part normal-to-dry (usually on the cheek area) and part oily (typically, the T-zone: forehead, nose and chin). With combination skin, the objective is to control oiliness without drying out the dryer areas of your face. Choose a mild cleanser for dry or normal skin, whichever is best suited to the cheek area of your face. Try Zotos UnSun Foaming Mousse Facial Cleanser. Wash gently in the morning and before bed, using a soft cloth or your finger tips. Rinse thoroughly and towel dry. After cleansing, apply a moisturizer, such as Purist Aloe and Paba All-Day Moisturizer or Zotos UnSun Facial Moisturizing Lotion, to the dryer areas of your face and a toner or astringent, such as Milk'N Honee Toner Lotion for Normal/Oily or Dry/Sensitive skin to the oilier areas of your face. If the T-zone is very oily, you may want to repeat using a toner or astringent during the day.

784. What causes acne?

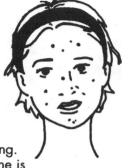

There are several factors that can contribute to breakouts: heredity; a fluctuation in the level of hormones caused by puberty, pregnancy or menstruation; improper cleansing and the use of incorrect skin care products; stress; and irritation caused by constant chafing. There is no proof that acne is caused by food products, but food allergies can cause rashes resembling acne.

785. I have moderate acne—small pimples and blackheads on my face. Is soap the best cleanser for my skin?

Many dermatologists believe that the best way to cleanse acne-prone skin is with a mild soapless or non-soap cleanser. Try Milk'N Honee Facial Wash for Acne-Prone Skin, a 100 percent non-soap with collagen-based protein cleanser and pH 5.5. Acne-prone skin should always be treated gently. Don't scrub your face with abrasive sponges or cleansers. Wash using gentle circular motions and lukewarm, not hot, water. Do not squeeze pimples! Squeezing can cause more skin eruptions and can cause scarring. To control pimples, follow cleansing with an acne-control product containing benzoyl peroxide, salicylic acid or alpha hydroxy acids. Try Freeman Professional's Aromesentials Alpha Hydroxy Toner.

786. I have sensitive, acne-prone skin. What is the most effective way to cleanse without irritating my skin?

Contrary to popular belief, it is not necessary to scrub acne-prone skin with harsh soaps or abrasive cleansers. Scrubbing can irritate your skin and cause acne to worsen. Gentle cleansing should be done with a mild, soap-less cleanser, such as Purist Aloe Vera and NaPCA Creamy Facial Wash. Wash with the finger tips and use lukewarm rather than hot water. Don't overdo it. Cleansing twice a day is adequate. Follow with a mild, medicated acne treatment product to help rid your skin of present pimples and prevent break-outs. If your skin is particularly sensitive or your acne is severe, consult a dermatologist.

787. I've tried every benzoyl peroxide acne product on the market without success. What should I do?

Although it is an effective acne treatment, benzoyl peroxide is not right for everyone, and not all acne can be effectively treated with over-the-counter products. Try other anti-acne ingredients available in over-the-counter products, such as salicylic acid, alpha hydroxy acids, sulfur and resorcinol. However, if your skin resists treatment, consult a dermatologist.

788. What are the benefits of products containing salicylic acid?

Salicylic acid (beta hydroxy acid) acts as a peeling agent and loosens debris from clogged pores. It is particularly helpful for blackheads. Check out Milk'N Honee Essential Day Moisturizer which contains salicylic acid.

789. What are blackheads?

Blackheads, like whiteheads, are a mixture of dead skin cells, oil and bacteria. When exposed to the oxygen in the air, a chemical reaction causes this mixture to darken.

F.Y. 👁 Skin Facts

The skin is the body's largest organ, measuring approximately two square yards and accounting for about 15 percent of the body's weight. Skin is thickest on the back, palms and the soles of the feet. The thinnest skin is on the eyelids. The body's skin serves several functions; it not only protects the inner body from the environment, it also expels waste and regulates body temperature. The skin is divided into three layers: the epidermis, the dermis and the subcutis.

- The subcutis is the fatty base layer that cushions your internal organs, conserves heat and serves as an energy reserve for the body.

- The dermis contains collagen and elastin, the complex proteins responsible for the support and elasticity of the skin. Collagen accounts for most of the weight and the strength of the dermis. When collagen sags, wrinkles occur. The dermis is where the sensory nerve endings are that allow you to feel pressure, vibration and pain. The skin's nutrition and oxygenation are supplied via tiny arteries, veins and capillaries that run through the dermis.

- The epidermis, the outermost layer of skin, is constantly undergoing a process of regeneration. New cells are formed in the bottom layer (basal layer) and over time move up through the epidermis until they reach the surface layer (stratum corneum) where they are shed. This cell turnover takes about one month. The stratum corneum is sometimes called the "acid mantle," because its pH is 5.5, or slightly acidic. The basal layer also contains the cells that produce melanin, the skin's pigment. The more melanin produced, the darker the skin color.

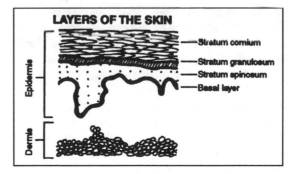

LAYERS OF THE SKIN

790. What is Retin-A?

One of the most effective topical anti-acne treatments, Retin-A is also called Vitamin A acid, Retinoic Acid, or Tretinoin. It is only available by prescription from a doctor. Retin-A accelerates cell turnover, speeding the production of new skin cells. This increased cell turnover helps clear up inflammatory acne lesions. More recently, Retin-A has become known for its effectiveness in treating wrinkles, typically the result of sun damage (photoaging).

791. How is Retin-A used?

Retin-A is a topical prescription medication that must be used only under the care of a physician. It is available in a cream, liquid or gel form and in several strengths. Typically it is applied to the skin as one would apply a moisturizer or cream.

792. If Retin-A is an acid, is it safe for your skin?

Retin-A is safe as long as it is used under the care of a physician. It is currently not available without a doctor's prescription.

793. I am an African-American woman with acne. Some of the products I've tried darken my skin. Are there special acne treatment guidelines for African-Americans?

Benzoyl peroxide, an effective acne treatment found in many over-the-counter acne products, can sometimes darken African-American skin. Retin-A, a prescription-only acne treatment, can sometimes lighten skin. Acne scarring also causes changes in pigmentation, so be espe-

cially gentle in washing and caring for deeply pigmented acne-prone skin. Do not squeeze pimples! Squeezing can cause scarring. When using acne treatments, start slowly to test for sensitivity and irritation. If acne or discoloration is severe, consult a dermatologist.

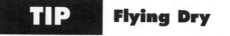

TIP **Flying Dry**

To keep skin hydrated in the drying atmosphere of an airplane cabin, moisturize your face well and be sure to drink plenty of water throughout the flight. Avoid such in-flight dehydrators as alcohol and salty nuts.

794. Why are toners or fresheners used?

Toning lotions—toners, fresheners and astringents—are designed to remove oil, to give skin a fresh, invigorated feeling, and to temporarily tighten pores. Toning products are generally used after or between facial cleansings and are helpful in removing excess oil from oily and combination skin types. There are two basic types: alcohol-based and alcohol-free. Because alcohol is drying to the skin, alcohol-based products are not recommended for normal-to-dry or sensitive skin. Some toning products formulated for acne-prone skin contain ingredients such as salicylic acid or resorcinol. Try Purist Water Lily Pore Lotion Astringent for oily or combination skin. For acne-prone skin, try Purist Antiseptic Clarifying Deep Cleansing Lotion. Alcohol-free toners and fresheners often contain humecants, such as glycerin, which attract and hold moisture, as well as botanical ingredients. For normal to dry skin, try Purist Camomile and NaPCA

Clarifying Toner or Milk'N Honee Toner Lotion for Dry, Sensitive Skin.

795. No matter what I do in the morning, by noon my skin feels oily. What can I do?

After cleansing your face in the morning, saturate a cotton square with toner or astringent formulated for oily skin. Try Milk'N Honee Toner Lotion for Normal to Oily Skin. Wipe the cotton pad across the oily areas of your face. Use an oil-free foundation and powder or gel blush. Dust your face lightly with translucent powder or set your makeup with translucent powder and a large puff. If your skin feels oily by midday, refresh your face with another application of toner. Tip: Fill a purse-size bottle with your toning product and carry a few quilted cotton pads. Finish with an oil-blotting pressed powder.

796. Lately my chin area has been breaking out. Could this be caused by the telephone?

Hands, sports equipment, clothing or even the telephone can induce acne mechanica, a form of acne caused by repeated rubbing or touching. Try to avoid touching the phone to your face. If your chin area tends to be oily, wipe the phone with a cleanser, such as Beauty Secrets Gel Guard Skin Sanitizer after using the it. Also, because phones are both touched and breathed upon by many people, bacteria can build up. Make sure the phone is cleaned frequently.

797. Are those pimples on my back and upper arms considered acne?

Acne may appear on the upper back, but those pimples on your upper arms may actually be an allergy or related to hay fever. Consult your dermatologist to determine the cause and need for a medicated moisturizer. Avoid scrubbing the area, as it could make the problem worse.

798. Can I wear makeup over acne products without aggravating my skin?

Yes. Makeup can easily be worn over acne treatments, but be sure to choose makeup products that are oil-free and noncomedegenic (non-clogging). Read labels carefully.

799. What is the purpose of exfoliating?

Exfoliation is the process of removing the dead cells on the top layer (stratum corneum) of your skin. To a lesser extent, exfoliation can help dislodge blackheads. The procedure is referred to as "exfoliation" because when a mild abrasive is used on the skin, the top layer of dead skin cells is shed or exfoliated. Exfoliators include everything from washcloths, buffing sponges, facial brushes and loofahs to cleansing grains, sloughing cleansers and scrubs (cleansers or moisturizers that contain abrasive particles or ingredients), to alpha hydroxy acid (AHA), benzoyl peroxide and salicylic acid formulas that exfoliate chemically. In moderation and performed gently, exfoliating can be beneficial for most skin types. Exfoliating stimulates circulation and leaves skin looking smoother, finer and clearer.

800. What type of exfoliating products are available?

There are facial scrub products formulated for every skin type, from oil-free products designed to remove excess oil, to oil-based scrubs intended to remove dead skin cells while replacing lost oil. Some scrub products to consider are Beauty Secrets Beauty Buff in Regular or Gentle, Gigi Loofah Complexion Disk, Purist Apricot and Kelp Facial Scrub, and Aromesentials Cherry Blossom and Almond Facial/Body Scrub. Remember: avoid abrasive products if you have acne. Scrubs are not effective on pimples and can irritate acne-prone skin, aggravating the condition.

801. What is meant by the term "cell renewal"?

The cells of the top layer of skin (epidermis) are in a constant process of regeneration or renewal. New cells are formed in the bottom (basal) layer of the epidermis and make their way to the skin's surface where they are shed or exfoliated. Shedding old skin cells stimulates the formation of new skin cells. Thus, products that exfoliate and remove old skin cells speed up the process of cell renewal.

802. Will a buffing sponge damage my skin?

Buffing sponges can be used safely if used

F.Y. **Identify Your Skin Type**

To properly care for your skin, you must first identify your skin type, since the products and methods of skin care you use should be tailored to your skin's level of moisture and sensitivity. Keep in mind that skin is affected by the environment. Sun, cold, wind, pollution, indoor heat and air conditioning all tend to be drying. Furthermore, skin changes as we age; it tends to be oilier during adolescence and dryer as we grow older.

To determine your skin type, wash your face with a mild soap and rinse thoroughly. Do not apply moisturizer. Several hours later, look at your skin in a magnifying mirror in bright, preferably natural, light.

- You have dry skin if:
  Skin appears dry and may be flaky with barely visible pores.

- You have normal skin if:
  Skin appears moist and smooth but not oily. Pores are visible but unclogged.

- You have oily skin if:
  Skin appears shiny with large, often clogged, pores.

- You have combination skin if:
  Cheeks are moist or even dry. The T-zone (nose, chin and forehead) appears oily with some clogged pores.

- You have sensitive skin if:
  Skin is easily irritated, whether dry, normal or oily. At times skin itches, burns or stings.

moderately—less than a minute—and gently, with very light pressure. Don't use a buffing sponge with an abrasive cleanser. If you have oily skin, you may want to exfoliate with a buffing sponge twice weekly. If your skin is normal to dry, once every week or two should be adequate. Buffing sponges may be too harsh for some skins. A soft washcloth or a scrub product formulated for dry skin may be better choices. Do not use a buffing sponge on pimples, acne or broken skin. Scrubbing worsens the problem.

803. What is gentler on the skin, buffing sponges or scrubs?

Because they are available in so many formulations, some scrubs may be gentler than buffing sponges. If gentleness is your concern, use very light pressure over a short duration. A soft washcloth or natural sea sponge, like Gigi Natural Sea Sponge, is also a gentle exfoliator.

804. Are there scrubs specially formulated for dry skin?

Yes. Most scrubs formulated for dry skin have a cream base. Use them with care—gently massaging for about 30 seconds. A weekly scrub with a product formulated for dry skin can leave dry skin soft and smooth. Try Milk'N Honee Facial Scrub.

805. Are facial scrubs beneficial for acne-prone skin?

Unless under the direction of a dermatologist, avoid facial scrubs if you have acne-prone skin. Scrubs and abrasives are not effective on pimples and can irritate acne and can actually promote, instead of prevent, flare-ups.

806. Will facial scrubs get rid of blackheads and whiteheads?

Although facial scrubs slough off old skin cells and leave skin smooth and clearer looking, they are less effective in eliminating blackheads and whiteheads. Better choices for this problem would be a topical gel or lotion containing salicylic acid, which loosens and softens clogged pores, or an alpha hydroxy acid product, which can help to unclog pores. Check out Purist Skin Therapy's Alpha Hydroxy skin care products.

807. Are facial scrubs containing natural ingredients, such as oatmeal or apricot seed, better than scrubs containing synthetic grains?

Some skin experts believe that man-made cleansing grains specifically designed for exfoliation are gentler on skin than the natural ingredients often used, such as crushed apricot kernels, walnut shells or pumice. Others believe that naturals are better. Try Aromesentials Sea Kelp and Mango Facial Scrub or Milk'N Honee Facial Scrub and see which works better for you. Oatmeal and cornmeal are gentler, natural ingredients that have long been used to exfoliate the skin. Whatever facial scrub you use, remember, don't overdo it. Keep scrubbing time under one minute and use light, circular strokes. Rinse well.

808. What are alpha hydroxy acids (AHAs)?

Alpha hydroxy acids, known as AHAs, are a group of several acids—including citric acid (from citrus fruits), lactic acid (from sour milk), glycolic acid (from sugar cane), tartaric acid (from aged wine) and malic acid (from

apples)—that bear chemical similarities. Although these ingredients occur naturally, they can also be formulated in the laboratory, as with most of the glycolic acids used today. AHAs affect the outermost layer of the skin (stratum corneum), causing dead skin cells (keratin cells) to lift off and separate from the underlying skin, revealing newer cells with a smoother look and texture. AHAs are also showing some effectiveness in reducing the fine wrinkling associated with aging. AHAs are available in cream, gel and lotion formulas at various prices. Purist Skin Therapy offers a complete alpha hydroxy skin care line that is economically priced. Other professional quality AHA lines include Aromesentials Alpha Hydroxy lotion, toner or soap or Jheri Redding's Milk'N Honee Facial Scrub, Facial Masque and Moisturizer or Zotos UnSun Reparative Age Control Creme and Facial Moisturizing Lotion.

809. Can AHAs benefit both dry and oily skin?

Yes. Alpha hydroxy acids exfoliate both dry and oily skins to produce smoother-textured, clearer-looking skin.

810. Can AHAs help improve acne?

AHAs have the benefit of being effective agents against acne because they can aid in unclogging pores and releasing whiteheads and blackheads. Try Milk'N Honee Facial Masque, Purist Skin Therapy Retexturizing Mask or Zotos UnSun Reparative Cleanser Mask. For severe or persistent acne, consult a dermatologist.

811. Are skin care products containing AHAs beneficial for mature skin?

Yes. The exfoliation caused by AHAs gives mature skin a clearer, fresher look. As we age, the cell renewal process tends to slow down. AHAs stimulate cell turnover. There is also some evidence that AHAs have an "anti-wrinkle effect" due to the acids' action on the dermal layer of the skin. Research in this area is ongoing.

812. What is the recommended percentage range of AHAs in over-the-counter skin care products?

Many strengths of AHAs are available in both over-the-counter skin care products and by pre-scription from a doctor. In over-the-counter skin care products, the percentage of AHAs ranges from 2.5% to products such as Purist Skin Therapy Overnight Age Complex containing 8%. Anything over a 10% concentration should be administered under a physician's guidance.

813. What level AHA should I choose?

Most women can benefit from using AHAs in over-the-counter skin care products if they choose products appropriate for their individual skin type. If skin is sensitive, start with a low percentage (2.5% to 5%) and work up to higher levels if your skin can tolerate it. Remember that any new skin care regime will not produce visible results for several weeks.

814. How often should AHAs be used?

Most over-the-counter AHA skin care products are designed to be used on a daily basis. If you've never used AHA products, start slowly. Because AHAs can irritate some skin, begin with a low percentage (2.5% to 5%) AHA product and use every other day. Increase usage to twice daily before trying a stronger formula. Let your own skin's response be your guide. Keep in mind that it may take three to four weeks to see the benefits of AHAs. Formulations stronger than 10% must be administered and monitored by a physician.

815. How should AHAs be applied?

Cleanse face first to remove surface oils that

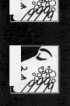

F.Y. Good Skin Sense

While the relative effectiveness of the ever-increasing proliferation of skin care products available is debatable, there are some basic truths of skin care, hazards to avoid and preventive measures we can take.

- **Sun Exposure**
  Sun exposure damages skin. It is the major cause of premature aging and can cause skin cancer. Sun damage is cumulative from childhood. Correct and appropriate use of sunscreen is the most effective preventive measure we can take.

- **Smoking and Alcohol**
  Smoking decreases the skin's oxygen intake and contributes to the breakdown of the collagen and elastin in the skin.

Furthermore, wrinkling of the upper lip is caused by repetitive puffing. For these, and other reasons, don't smoke. Alcohol expands the blood vessels and can cause broken capillaries.

- **Makeup**
  Makeup should be thoroughly removed at night to prevent clogged pores and those "raccoon eyes." Makeup should be tailored to skin type. Using the wrong formulation can cause skin to break out. Makeup applicators should be washed and regularly replaced to prevent the spread of bacteria.

- **Gentle Treatment**
  All skin should be treated gently, but

particularly acne-prone skin. Squeezing pimples and scrubbing too hard can cause scarring or break-outs.

- **Stress, Sleep and Diet**
  Stress and sleep deprivation are responsible for dark undereye circles as well as acne eruptions. Get plenty of "beauty sleep" and try a massage to relax and relieve tense muscles. Poor nutrition shows in the condition of the skin. Eat a balanced diet and include foods high in vitamins A, C and E. These antioxidant vitamins help fight free radicals released by pollution and other elements in our environment that damage skin cells.

could interfere with AHA penetration. For dry or normal skin, try a moisturizing formula containing AHAs, such as Purist Skin Therapy Day Moisture Cream, Milk'N Honee Day Moisturizer for Dry, Sensitive Skin, or Zotos UnSun Facial Moisturizing Lotion. For oily skin, try Milk'N Honee Day Moisturizer for Normal to Oily Skin. Apply just enough to cover the skin and gently rub it in. Avoid the sensitive eye area.

816. When I tried a skin care product containing AHAs, my skin became red and irritated. Should I discontinue using it?

Some skin redness and irritation is normal with AHAs. This effect usually diminishes with continued use of AHAs, as the skin develops a tolerance. Whether or not you will experience side effects from a skin care product containing AHA depends on the strength of the AHA concentration. For this reason, it is advisable to start with a low concentration (2.5% to 3%) and increase slowly. Some skin care experts advise waiting 15 minutes after cleansing to avoid irritation. Keep in mind that irritation could also be the result of allergies to other ingredients in the product. If irritation persists, discontinue use.

817. What are the benefits of a facial mask?

Cleansing masks leave skin smooth and glowing. Moisturizing masks or cream masks are intended to soften dry skin.

818. What is a "deep-cleansing" mask? How often should they be used?

Deep-cleansing masks remove excess oil and dirt along with dead skin cells to give the skin a smoother texture and healthy glow. There are two types of masks: wash-off (usually clay- or mud-based) and peel-off (a liquid film which dries to a peelable sheet). Because clay masks are effective oil absorbers, they're best for oily or combination skins. If your skin is oily, you may use a clay mask as often as once a week. Women with combination skin may want to apply a mask to the T-zone area only. If your skin is dry to normal, don't use a mask more than once or twice a month. And if your skin is very dry or sensitive, avoid drying, clay-based masks. Don't apply any mask near your eyes; masks are too drying for the delicate eye area. For oily or combination skin, try Purist Clay and Mineral Skin Purifying Mask. For normal skin, try Aromesentials Peppermint Rosemary Facial Mask. For dry skin, try Zotos UnSun Reparative Cleansing Mask.

819. Should I apply a moisturizer after a deep-cleansing mask?

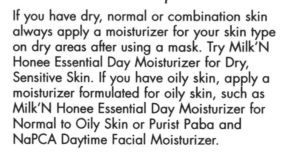

If you have dry, normal or combination skin always apply a moisturizer for your skin type on dry areas after using a mask. Try Milk'N Honee Essential Day Moisturizer for Dry, Sensitive Skin. If you have oily skin, apply a moisturizer formulated for oily skin, such as Milk'N Honee Essential Day Moisturizer for Normal to Oily Skin or Purist Paba and NaPCA Daytime Facial Moisturizer.

820. Can dry skin benefit from a facial mask?

If you have dry skin with barely visible pores, avoid a drying, clay-based mask and instead try a moisturizing mask, such as Purist Aloe Vera Face Pack or Blue Velvet Face Mask.

821. What does a salon facial consist of?

A professional salon facial leaves your skin soft, clean and clear and your body feeling relaxed and pampered. Facial treatments vary from salon to salon. Typically during a one hour session, the esthetician examines and evaluates your skin's type and condition. Next, she cleanses, massages and moisturizes your skin before giving it a gentle steaming to open pores. The facialist then unclogs pores and may apply a toner or astringent. A facial mask formulated for your skin type is applied and left on approximately 10 to 15 minutes, then removed. A paraffin mask may then be applied after the first mask to further smooth the skin. After the skin is cleaned of all products and sprayed with a mist or freshener, the esthetician gently blots the skin and applies a moisturizer. Some facialists also give an upper-shoulder massage to relieve tension. If you are having your first facial, alert the esthetician before she begins. Skin that isn't used to being constantly touched can become over-stimulated, leading to a later breakout. Note: It is normal for skin to look flushed immediately after a facial.

822. What is the best way to care for my skin between salon facials?

Stick with a regular skin care regime of cleansing, toning and moisturizing, based on your skin type. Treat your skin gently; don't poke and prod! Wear a sunscreen with at least an SPF 15 from April to November. If your skin is fair, wear sunscreen year-round. Try Zotos UnSun Moisturizing Lotion SPF 15.

823. How often should I have a salon facial?

Have a salon facial every 4-6 weeks to maintain healthy skin. Some people prefer to have facials two times a month, usually because they have a recurring skin problem, like acne. If on a budget, every three months is adequate, but it depends on the condition of your skin. For best results, estheticians recommend having a salon facial once a month.

824. What are moisturizers? Do all skin types need moisturizing?

The principal ingredients in most moisturizers are water and emollients (animal, vegetable or petroleum-based oils) which act as a barrier to moisture loss. Oil-free moisturizers contain humectants (such as glycerin, propylene glycol and lactic acid) that work by drawing water into the outermost layer of the skin (stratum corneum). Some moisturizers contain both emollients and humectants. Facial moisturizers designed for day use are usually of a lighter consistency than facial night creams or eye creams. Moisturizers are also formulated by skin type: more emollient formulas for dry skin; oil-free, noncomedegenic formulas for oily skins. Although people with oily skin may not need a facial moisturizer, because there are many contributors to skin moisture loss—age, heat, cold, wind, sun, as well as indoor heating and cooling—most people benefit from using a moisturizer.

825. What is the difference between moisturizing creams and lotions?

Creams are thicker and heavier in texture and contain more emollients than water. Lotions are more liquid and lighter in texture and generally contain more water than emollients.

826. My skin is dry, yet I hate the greasy look of heavy creams. What can I use?

Try using a moisturizing lotion, like Aromesentials Butter Rose & Chamomile Facial Moisturizer. Apply it all over your face and neck after cleansing and rinsing your face. Reapply during the day, as needed, and at night before bed. You may also want to treat yourself to a salon facial paraffin treatment or a hydration mask, like Purist Aloe Vera Face Pack.

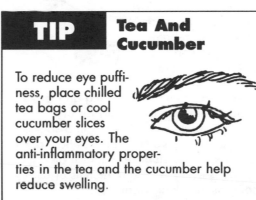

TIP — **Tea And Cucumber**

To reduce eye puffiness, place chilled tea bags or cool cucumber slices over your eyes. The anti-inflammatory properties in the tea and the cucumber help reduce swelling.

---

827. I use a cleansing cream to remove makeup from my dry skin. Should I apply a moisturizer afterward?

Yes, but make sure you remove all traces of cleansing cream first. While you may think that the light residue of a cleansing cream would be fine for very dry skin, some cleansing creams also contain soap or detergent ingredients which can be irritating if left on the skin. Try Purist Skin Therapy Perfecting Cleanser or Purist Fresh Lemon Deep Pore Cleansing Cream. If removing your cleansing cream with tissues irritates your skin, try gently wiping it off with a lukewarm washcloth. Apply moisturizer, such as Purist Aloe Vera and Paba All Day Moisture Cream, immediately afterward.

828. I have oily skin but sometimes it feels dry on the surface. How can I add moisture without oil?

You may have combination skin: dry on the cheeks and oily in the T-zone and around the hairline. Apply an oil-free, noncomedegenic (non-clogging) moisturizer on any dry areas of your face after cleansing in the morning and at night. Or, you may be overusing an alcohol astringent and stripping the top layer of moisture while prompting the skin to produce more oil. Discontinue using your alcohol-based toner and try a non-alcohol formula like Milk'N Honee Tonic Lotion. You may want to try a product containing an alpha hydroxy acid, such as Aromesentials Alpha Hydroxy Toner, to help gently slough off dry skin cells.

829. My acne-prone skin often feels dry. How can I moisturize my skin without causing it to break out?

This dryness could be a result of using benzoyl peroxide or other ingredients used for treating acne. It also could be the result of washing or scrubbing your skin with an abrasive sponge or with a cleanser that is too harsh. Remember, acne-prone skin should always be treated gently; scrubbing will aggravate, not improve, acne. Try using a mild nonsoap cleanser, such as Milk'N Honee Facial Wash for Skin with

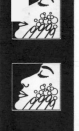

Acne Problems, and apply a light, oil-free, non-comedegenic (non-clogging) moisturizer, such as Milk'N Honee Essential Day Moisturizer for Normal Skin, to any dry areas. If you are under a doctor's treatment, consult your physician.

830. My skin doesn't feel dry. Should I use a moisturizer anyway?

If your skin is normal or oily, you may not need to use a moisturizer. However, if you are regularly exposed to harsh weather conditions (sun, wind or cold), wear a moisturizing sunscreen, such as Milk'N Honee Essential Day Moisturizer for Normal to Oily Skin. If your skin is subjected to indoor climate control (heating or air-conditioning) or if you frequently travel by air, a moisturizer, such as Aromesentials Alpha Hydroxy Lotion, is recommended. Apply after cleansing in the morning and at night.

831. Should I use the same facial moisturizer in the summer as in the winter?

Although in summer our faces tend to be more exposed to the elements, most people tend to have dryer skin during the winter months due to the combination of the outdoor elements and indoor heating. Unless your skin is oily, you may want to use a slightly heavier moisturizing product—a cream instead of a lotion—during the winter. Try Purist Aloe Vera and Paba All Day Moisture Cream. In summer, or on the slopes, use a sunscreen as well as a moisturizer or a moisturizer containing sun protection, such as Milk'N Honee Liposome Hyper Moisturizer Face Cream with SPF 4. Make sure you check the SPF factor on the package. For outdoor sports, SPF 15 is widely recommended by dermatologists for longer protection. Try Zotos UnSun Moisturizing Lotion with SPF 15.

832. Do I need to use a special eye cream? What are the benefits?

The skin around the eyes is the thinnest on your body. Eye creams are generally moisturizers that are specially formulated for this very sensitive area. They are intended to moisturize and soften the skin as well as improve the appearance of wrinkles. Try Purist Anti-Wrinkle Eye & Throat Cream. Other eye creams are formulated to reduce puffiness or to temporarily firm the skin around the eyes and reduce "bags," such as Claudia Stevens Under Eye Gel. Be sure to read the label carefully.

TIP — **Bain de Bacteria**

Beware, bacteria loves the warm and moist environment of a bathroom and can breed in loofahs and other bath sponges. Be sure to rinse sponges well after using and leave them where they can easily air dry. Once a week, soak sponges in a solution of bleach and water (1 part bleach to 10 parts water) to sterilize. Replace all bath sponges every couple of months or as soon as they look worn.

---

833. Can moisturizers or skin creams prevent premature aging?

Moisturizers and skin creams can't slow, stop or reverse the aging process. However, they are important in maintaining soft, smooth, supple skin. To prevent premature aging, always use SPF 15 sun protection, such as Zotos UnSun Moisturizing Lotion SPF 15.

Most dermatologists agree that "photoaging" is responsible for as much as 70% to 90% of the skin damage—wrinkling, sagging and discoloration—we associate with aging.

834. What is the difference between day moisturizers and night creams? Do I need a special cream at night?

Daytime moisturizers are usually lighter in consistency and quickly disappear into the skin, creating a suitable base for makeup. Night creams are generally heavier, cream formulations. Whether you use a special cream at night is really a matter of personal preference. Some women prefer the benefit of a thicker emollient before bed when makeup application is not a consideration. Try Purist Active Nutrisom Age-Control Cream. Other women take advantage of night creams with higher concentrations (8-10%) of alpha hydroxy acids designed to exfoliate the skin. Try Purist Skin Therapy Overnight Age Management Complex.

835. Will products containing AHAs remove age spots?

AHAs help to slough off the top layer of skin cells, and when applied in higher concentration, can improve superficial age spots. However, there is a limit to how deep the AHAs can peel the skin, therefore deeper pigmentation may not show significant improvement with the use of AHAs. For best results, consult your dermatologist.

836. What are "free radicals" and "antioxidants"?

Free radicals (oxidants) are unstable oxygen molecules that damage skin cells. Free radicals are caused by pollution, ultraviolet light, environmental conditions and some foods. Antioxidants—including vitamin E, betacarotene (vitamin A precursor) and vitamin C—may help prevent free radical damage when taken orally as vitamins. While some cosmetic companies have introduced antioxidants into their products, it's not firmly established whether they are effective when applied topically.

837. Is my body skin the same type as my facial skin?

While the skin is one organ, because certain parts of your body vary in thickness or are more exposed to environmental factors, the skin on your body can sometimes seem like a patchwork of different skin types. Certain body parts, such as feet, hands and elbows, tend to be dryer than the rest of your body. Other body areas, such as the shoulders, back and chest can be oily or acne-prone in people with oily or acne-prone facial skin. Skin that is usually not exposed to the elements can be more sensitive to sun exposure and other environmental factors and often feels and reacts differently than the skin on your face.

838. What is aromatherapy?

Aromatherapy is a term that refers to the therapeutic use of botanical essences. When used in aromatic baths, massage or skin care, the essential oils derived from a variety of herbs, flowers, bushes and trees are said to stimulate, exhilarate, relax, calm or soothe, depending upon the essences used. Although the term aromatherapy was coined in the

1920s, the medicinal and cosmetic use of plants and their essences dates back to the ancient Egyptians and has evolved to regain attention and respect today.

839. Is it better to bathe or to shower?

Whether you bathe or shower is a matter of personal preference. Bathing tends to be more relaxing. For an aromatherapy bath, try Freeman Professional Aromesentials Mango & Blueberry Bath Foam: mango soothes and revitalizes while blueberry calms and tones. Or, consider Aromesentials Raspberry and Calendula Bath Foam: raspberry relaxes while calendula soothes. Bathe in warm water and don't stay in the tub too long. Prolonged soaking in hot water can actually rob the skin's moisture. Showering is more stimulating. Use a bath gel with a natural or mesh sponge, such as Gigi Natural Loofa or Body Image Netted Beauty Sponge, to exfoliate the skin and stimulate circulation. Try Freeman Professional Aromesentials Lemongrass and Kiwi Fruit Bath Gel formulated to energize and moisturize the skin.

840. What type of cleanser should I use on my body? Is bath or shower gel better than soap?

Soap or gel is a matter of personal preference. Unlike basic soaps, nonsoap bath or shower gels do not react with hard water to produce "soap scum residue." Gels lather easily and can be used with natural or mesh sponges. Try Freeman Professional Aromesentials Peach Tree and Gardenia Bath Gel, designed to exhilarate, condition and soften skin. If you prefer a bar soap, try

Aromesentials Alpha-Hydroxy Kiwi & Bilberry Soap, or Milk'N Honee Beauty Bar.

841. Are there special bath products for sore, aching muscles?

Mineral salt baths have long been recognized as effective alleviators of body aches. Try Batherapy®, a concentrated bath salt containing many natural minerals similar to those found in hot springs and spas.

842. I have dry skin. What afterbath product will soothe and soften my skin?

Because of its relatively high vitamin content, sweet almond oil is considered particularly nourishing for dry skin. Freeman Aromesentials Sweet Almond Oil & Sunflower After-Bath Silkener leaves your body soft and smooth without any greasy residue. Aloe vera has also long been recognized as a skin soother and acts as a humectant to keep moisture in the skin. Try Palm Beach Skin Saver, Triple Lanolin Aloe Vera Lotion, or Malibu Tan Pure Aloe Gel.

843. What kinds of services are offered at a day spa?

Treatments and charges vary greatly from spa to spa but here are some of the services frequently offered. Facials usually include skin analysis, clarification, cleansing, exfoliation, mask, toning and hydration; facial paraffin treatments are also frequently offered. Body treatments may include sauna, whirlpool, jet bath, steamroom, massage, mud bath, salt scrub, seaweed body wraps, clay or herbal body masks, reflexology and waxing. Day spas also usually offer nail services, such as manicures, pedicures and paraffin treatments.

844. What are facial paraffin treatments?

Similar to the paraffin hand and foot wraps, facial paraffin treatments are intended to moisturize and soften. An aesthetician applies a moisturizing treatment and then coats the skin with warm paraffin which is left on the face for 10 to 15 minutes. The paraffin's warmth causes the pores to open, allowing moisturizers to penetrate more easily. When removed, the paraffin takes old skin cells with it, leaving the skin silky smooth and soft.

845. What is a "body mask"?

Similar to a facial mask, a body mask is intended to detoxify and refine the skin. After you spend a few minutes in a steamroom, a clay-based mask is applied over all or certain areas of the body. These masks can be formulated for different skin types and purposes and can incorporate herbs or other botanicals and their essences. The mask is left on the skin for about 10 to 20 minutes before being rinsed off. A moisturizer is then applied.

846. Which spa services are therapeutic and which are simply relaxing?

All spa services are intended to relax and refresh. They can be great anecdotes to stress. A massage can relax tight muscles, relieving back and shoulder pain. A facial can help

relax tightened facial muscles. People come to a spa to feel pampered, to be beautified and to go away refreshed, relaxed and glowing.

847. How can I create an at-home spa?

Give yourself several hours without interruption. Take a warm bath with a deliciously scented bath gel, such as Aromesentials Peach Tree & Gardenia. Use a loofah or net sponge to stimulate and exfoliate your skin. After your bath, moisturize your body with a softening formula, such as Milk'N Honee Body Milk. Apply a facial mask designed for your skin's needs. For oily skin, try Purist Fresh Lemon Face Pac. For combination or normal skin, try Purist Mint Magic or Mud Miracle. For dry skin, try Purist Aloe Vera Face Pack or Zotos UnSun Reparative Cleansing Mask. Play your favorite soothing music, place a slice of cucumber over each eye, apply handcream, such as Milk'N Honee Hand & Body Cream, slip on White Cotton Beauty Gloves, and lie down for 10 to 15 minutes. Wash off the mask and apply a moisturizer, such as Aromesentials Alpha Hydroxy Lotion. For oily skin, use a non-alcohol-based toner, such as Aromesentials Kiwi & Bilberry Toner. Finish with an energizing pedicure, ending up with a cooling peppermint foot gel, like Perfect Feel Icy Foot Gel.

848. What are the best exfoliators for the body?

Take your pick from a whole range of body exfoliators. Mechanical exfoliators include a range of washcloths, natural and net sponges, bath brushes as well as cleansing grains and scrubs. Chemical exfoliators include a variety of alpha hydroxy acid products and body scrubs.

849. What is a loofah? How is it used?

A loofah is a natural sponge made from a loofah plant, sometimes made into a cloth or mitt. Because of its fibrous texture, a loofah is used to exfoliate the skin, i.e., slough off dead skin cells.

850. What is the difference between using a loofah and body cleansing grains?

Both exfoliate. A loofah works because of its texture. Body cleansing grains contain granules which when rubbed on the skin "polish" the body instead of washing it. Try body cleansing grains such as Aromesentials Cherry Blossom and Almond Face and Body Scrub or Zotos UnSun Gentle Exfoliating Cleansing Lotion.

851. Is there a difference between the natural sponges used by spas and the synthetic sponges I find in the drugstore?

Natural sponges are more durable than synthetic fibers, which is why you may find them at spas. They will hold up better over time. Try Gigi's Natural Sea Sponge.

852. Are products for the body containing AHAs different from formulas for the face?

Body care products, such as skin care lotion

and body bath gels containing AHAs, typically contain a lower concentration of AHAs due to the potential for skin sensitivity.

853. In winter I get little white bumps on my arms. What are they and what can I do about them?

Those bumps are probably dry skin that is stuck to the hair follicle. Exfoliating with a scrub product or sloughing sponge should solve the problem. Try Aromesentials Cherry Blossom and Almond Face and Body Scrub.

854. I have dark African-American skin, but my knees and elbows often look ashy. What can I do?

Try using an alpha hydroxy acid in a moisturizing formula like Purist Skin Therapy Hand & Body Lotion. It exfoliates the dry, surface skin to prevent the ashy appearance.

855. Should everyone moisturize after bathing?

If you have oily skin, it may not be necessary to use a moisturizer after bathing. But most people, especially those with dry and sensitive skin, can benefit from using a moisturizer.

856. Should I apply body creams in the morning and at night?

Generally, a body lotion or cream should be applied after bathing or showering, whether in the morning or at night. However, if you have flaky, dry skin or if you have been in the sun, it is beneficial to use body cream twice daily.

857. Should I use a different body cream in winter and summer?

Body creams and lotions are available in many formulations, but generally, body creams tend to be thicker in consistency and contain more emollients than lotions. Let the condition of your skin guide you. If your skin is dry and chapped from the cold of winter, a soothing cream, such as Milk'N Honee Hand and Body Cream or Queen Helene Cocoa Butter Creme helps. In the heat of summer, a lighter lotion moisturizes without leaving you feeling greasy. Try Milk'N Honee Body Milk or MRX Hydrating Lotion.

858. What is the best softener for the hands?

For smoothness and deep moisturizing, try a salon paraffin treatment that softens skin and cuticles with moisturizing oils. For daily use, try a moisturizing lotion like Skin Saver Aloe Vera Lotion, Vienna Triple Lanolin Hand and Body Lotion or Purist Skin Therapy Hand and Body Lotion for extra protection.

859. What is the best way to remove calluses and rough, dry skin from my feet?

Try Perfect Feet Sloughing Lotion or Aromesentials Tootsies Foot Scrub to remove dry skin and calluses. Follow with Perfect Feet Icy Foot Gel or Tootsies Peppermint Foot Lotion to energize and revitalize.

860. Is there a safe level for tanning?

We may wish for a "healthy tan," but there is no such thing as safe tanning. Exposure to ultraviolet light damages skin cells' genetic material and can contribute to skin cancer formation. Sun damage is cumulative: exposure to ultraviolet light during childhood will increase the risk of developing skin cancer in later years. However, it's never too late to begin using sunscreen to inhibit further sun damage.

861. What is "photoaging"?

"Photoaging" refers to the skin damage often associated with aging but actually incurred through sun exposure. Exposure to ultraviolet light causes the skin to thicken, resulting in a "leathery" appearance due to damage to the skin's collagen and elastin proteins. Sunlight also promotes broken blood vessels and discoloration of the skin. Sun damaged skin also tends to be dry and rougher in texture.

862. What is meant by "UVA" and "UVB"?

The sun emits several different types of radiation in addition to the visible light that we see. Ultraviolet A (UVA) and ultraviolet B (UVB) are two important types of invisible light that are potentially dangerous to your skin and are responsible for tanning and burning. Burning rays are more typical in the UVB range, but both promote photo-damage and the potential for skin cancer.

863. Do tanning salons provide a safer tan?

No. Since the early 1980s, when tanning salons were promoted as a safer alternative to sun exposure, it has become apparent that UVA light—typically the tanning salon's source of light—is damaging to the skin. It is now known that both UVB and UVA light can cause burning, photoaging and the skin changes associated with skin cancer. As of September 1986, the FDA required manufacturers of tanning devices to apply a warning label on all machines.

864. Why are some people more sensitive to sun exposure than others?

Sensitivity to sun damage depends on how much melanin (pigment) is produced within your skin: the less melanin, the greater the sensitivity to sun exposure. Differences in skin color between individuals or races are due to how much melanin is produced within the skin. Remember that only natural pigmentation is protective against sun damage; suntanned skin may prevent you from burning, but it does not provide protection from sun damage.

865. Are blondes more susceptible to photoaging?

Yes. The lack of skin pigment in blondes and redheads with fair skin leaves the underlying collagen in the skin more susceptible to the sun's damaging rays. While there are individual variations and exceptions, people of Celtic, Scandinavian or northern European descent tend to be the most sensitive to sun damage because they have the least melanin in their skin. People with Mediterranean backgrounds—Italian, Spaniard and Greek—are somewhat less sensitive. People of Asian and Hispanic heritage are moderately sensitive and those of African descent are the least sensitive to sun damage.

866. Do all suntan lotions contain sunscreen?

No! Although people have become more aware of the dangers of sun exposure, many tanning lotions, creams and oils are designed to promote tanning and do not provide protection from sun damage. Be sure to check the label for the SPF.

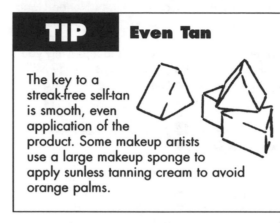

TIP **Even Tan**

The key to a streak-free self-tan is smooth, even application of the product. Some makeup artists use a large makeup sponge to apply sunless tanning cream to avoid orange palms.

867. What does SPF mean?

SPF stands for "sun protection factor." SPF ratings range from a base of 2 to a peak of 50, providing the strongest protection. Most dermatologists believe that SPF 15 is adequate protection. To estimate how long you can stay in the sun without burning, multiply the number of minutes it normally takes your skin to turn red by the SPF. For example, if your unprotected skin begins to redden in 10 minutes, an SPF of 15 will give you 150 minutes (2 1/2 hours) of sun protection (10 minutes x SPF 15=150).

868. How can I know what level of sun protection is right for me?

Generally, the lighter your skin, the higher SPF you'll need. SPF 2-6 provides minimal

protection for skin that is deeply pigmented and rarely burns; 6-8 gives moderate protection to skin that tans well and seldom burns; 10-15 is appropriate for people with medium, fair or sun-sensitive skin that tans minimally; 15-plus is necessary for people with very fair, sun-sensitive skin that burns easily and rarely tans.

869. My skin is dark olive. It tans easily and never burns. Do I need a sunscreen?

If you have olive skin, you are less likely to burn, but exposure to ultraviolet rays can still cause damage, including photoaging and skin cancer. Try Milk'N Honee Essential Day Moisturizer with SPF 4.

870. I'm African-American. Do I need a sunscreen?

While deeply pigmented skin is more resistant to sun damage than light skin, there is a great variation in skin tone among African-American women. Many dermatologists believe that black women should not risk the possibility of photoaging from sun exposure and recommend wearing sunscreen. Try a lower SPF formula, such as Purist Paba and NaPCA Daytime Moisturizer.

871. My lips are very sun sensitive. What is the best way to protect them?

Lips are particularly prone to sun damage. Use a product such as Beyond Belief Lip Balm that is designed to provide long-lasting sun protection.

872. Does where you live affect your susceptibility to damage from sun exposure?

If you live in an area of year-round sun exposure or at a high altitude where sunlight is more intense, you may sustain more damage due to sun exposure. If you live in such an area, be vigilant about applying sun protection with SPF 15 or higher, such as Zotos UnSun Moisturizing SPF 15 or Malibu Tanning Lotion SPF 15.

873. What is the safest time of day to be in the sun?

The sun's rays are most intense during the warmer half of the year. While sun damage can occur any time of day, avoid exposure when the sun is strongest—between the hours of 10 a.m. and 3 p.m. Water, sand and concrete reflect sunlight, intensifying its harmful effects. And remember, cloud cover is no protection from ultraviolet rays.

874. Which is best, alcohol-based, oil-based or cream-based sunscreen?

Sunscreens which are alcohol-based are better suited to oily or acne-prone skin; cream- or oil-based sunscreens are better for dry skin.

875. When and how should I apply sunscreen?

Apply sunscreen at least 30 minutes before going outdoors. Apply it liberally and be sure to cover all exposed areas including the backs of the knees, the tips of the ears and the tops of the feet.

876. How often should sunscreen be reapplied?

To ensure constant protection, reapply sunscreen after swimming or other physical activity and at regular intervals to be sure that perspiration doesn't leave you unprotected. Remember that reapplying sunscreen does not make it safer to stay in the sun longer, it just reestablishes the protection you have already applied.

877. What is the difference between a sunscreen and a sun block? Is it possible to burn while using a sunblock?

A chemically-based sunscreen contains one of several ingredients that absorb most of the ultraviolet rays, prolonging the time in which skin can be exposed to sunlight without burning. A sunblock is a physical sunscreen, i.e., a barrier against the ultraviolet rays of the sun. Sunblocks are available in creams or ointments containing titanium dioxide or the familiar white zinc oxide. If applied correctly, completely covering an area, such as the nose or lips, sunblocks are very effective in preventing sunburn. Because of their thick, greasy consistency they are inappropriate for oily skin types.

878. Can I use the same sunscreen on my face and on my body?

You can use the same formula or you can use two different ones. If your skin is oily, combination or acne prone, you will want an oil-free formula for your face, but you may want a more moisturizing lotion sunscreen for your body. Try UnSun Moisturizing Lotion SPF 15 for your face and Malibu Tanning Lotion SPF 15 for your body.

879. What is the difference between waterproof and water-resistant sunscreens? Do waterproof sunscreens last longer?

Because the sun's rays are not only reflected off water, but can also pass through it up to three feet, wearing sunscreen in the water—especially while snorkeling close to the water's surface—is very important. Water-resistant formulas stand up to water better than regular sunscreens. However, waterproof sunscreens are formulated to last twice as long as water-resistant formulas. To ensure continued protection, reapply after each swim.

880. I'm planning a honeymoon that will take us to several different locations. Can I wear a sunscreen with the same SPF level everywhere we go?

You many need an SPF 15 for a day on the slopes, a waterproof SPF 15 while waterskiing, and a lower SPF 8 when out shopping and sightseeing. However, if you choose to bring only one sunscreen, or if your skin is fair and very sun sensitive, opt for using an SPF 15 or higher.

881. Do I need a special sunscreen when I ski or play outdoor sports?

Because snow, sand, water, concrete and other surfaces on which people play or engage in outdoor sports are highly reflective and intensify the sun's rays, it is particularly important to wear an SPF 15 or higher sunscreen. Additionally, if your lips are particularly sensitive to sun damage, you may want to

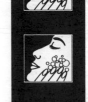

use a sun protection product that is designed for the lips. Try At One Lip Moisturizer.

882. Will a beach umbrella protect me from the sun?

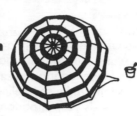

Because both sand and water reflect the sun's rays, sitting under an umbrella or in any shady location, does not necessarily keep you from getting a sunburn.

883. My skin is fair and dry. What type of sunscreen should I use?

For skin that is light in color and dry in texture, use an SPF 15 or higher sunscreen in a cream, rather than an alcohol-based formula. Read the label to make certain that the sunscreen protects against both UVB an UVA rays. Try Malibu Tanning Lotion SPF 15. Don't confuse cream-based sunscreens with suntan creams or oils without sun protection. Baby oil, coconut oil or cocoa butter are only lubricants and promote, rather than prevent sunburn.

884. My skin is oily. What type of sunscreen should I use?

For oily skin, use an alcohol-based, non-comedegenic sunscreen.

885. Is it true that sun exposure is good for acne-prone skin?

Although a suntan may mask blemished skin, sun exposure does not clear up acne and may even cause acne-prone skin to break out after exposure. Additionally, some women, especially those in their 20s or 30s, may have acne eruptions from exposure to the sun—especially if suntanning oils have been used.

886. Sunscreens irritate my sensitive skin. What can I do?

Check the ingredients in the sunscreen you are using. You may be allergic to PABA, an effective sunscreen ingredient. Look for a PABA-free sunscreen. Additionally, if you are allergic to hair dyes, avoid sunscreens containing PABA, since cross-reactivity can occur between PABA and an ingredient contained in most permanent hair dyes. Some women report burning and itching from high SPF sunscreens, but can tolerate lower concentrations.

887. Do lipsticks and foundations containing sunscreen offer enough protection?

Any cosmetic product containing sunscreen will have its SPF listed on the package. While many cosmetics now contain some level of sunscreen, be sure to check the package to make sure the product contains an adequate level of protection. SPF 15 is generally recommended by dermatologists for any facial application. When using a foundation with sunscreen be sure to cover your entire face, your neck and ears. Remember that these products are not waterproof; perspiration and water remove them.

888. Does sun exposure cause "age" spots?

"Age" spots are the flat spots often known as "liver" spots. These have nothing to do with your liver and may have received their name due to their light brown pigmentation. Typically seen in exposed areas of the face, back of hands and arms, they are the result of accumulated sun damage. In most cases they are harmless and possess no malignant potential. Age spots may be treated with chemical peels or skin care creams which contain AHAs or Retin-A.

889. Does sun exposure cause freckles?

Yes, sun exposure can cause freckles and other skin pigment changes.

890. What is self-tanning? Is it safe?

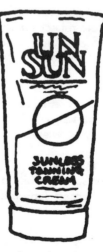

Self-tanning products contain the chemical dihydroxyacetone (DHA), an ingredient that has long been FDA approved as a food colorant. When applied to the skin, it reacts with the proteins and amino acids in the skin's surface layer, and produces a brown skin tone. Today's self-tanning products have improved color and odor. Test the product first on the inside of your arm to be sure you like the results. Remember, although self-tanners give you the look of a tan, they do not provide sun protection unless there is an SPF rating on the package.

891. What are bronzers? Are they different from self-tanners?

Bronzers contain water soluble pigment that is applied to the skin. Bronzers can be washed off easily and are a more temporary, cosmetic approach. Bronzing powders can be brushed on, much like blusher, with a large powder brush. Use a very light touch.

892. How can I apply a self-tanning product to ensure even color?

Even application is critical to achieving an even tan. Since most formulas disappear into the skin right away, it's sometimes hard to know exactly how much you've applied until the color develops. Dry skin tends to absorb more formula leading to streaks. For best results, exfoliate and shower to smooth and hydrate skin before applying a tanning product. Try Zotos UnSun Gentle Exfoliating Cleansing Lotion—it cleans, moisturizes and prepares skin for sunless tanning.

893. Which type of self-tanner is easiest to apply: a lotion, a gel or a spray?

This is more a matter of personal preference. Some people find massaging a cream or lotion over the body easier; others find sprays quick and convenient, especially for legs. Keep in mind that the objective is even application of the product to ensure an even tan, so use the method that you feel most comfortable with.

894. How can I avoid orange palms caused by self-tanning products?

To avoid color developing on the palms of your hands, scrub them with a nail brush immediately after applying a tanning product.

895. Why do self-tanners have such an unpleasant odor?

The odor is not in the product itself, but in the reaction of the product with the skin. Many manufacturers have found a way to eliminate the offensive smell. Try UnSun Sunless Tanning System.

896. Do I need to use separate self-tanning products on my face and my body?

It's not necessary to use separate products. Both UnSun Sunless Tanning System and Malibu Tan Sunless Tanning Lotion can be used on both your face and body.

897. Are there any secrets to applying self-tanning lotion to the face?

Work in small sections, massaging the self-tanner into the skin to cover evenly. Don't leave a chin line, and cover your neck, too.

For a hint of color, some makeup artists dilute self-tanning cream with a moisturizer. If the result is too light, reapply.

898. Can self-tanning products be worn in the sun? Do I need to wear sunscreen?

The "tan" you receive with a self-tanning product is no protection against the sun's ultraviolet rays, so you do need to wear sunscreen with a self-tanning product, unless the self-tanner displays a sun protection factor (SPF) on the package.

899. Do day spas offer self-tanning application treatments?

Yes. Many spas offer all-over self-tanner application. If you have a brand you like best, bring it with you.

900. How long will my "tan-in-a-tube" last?

Your tan should last 3 to 5 days, until the surface of the skin has naturally shed.

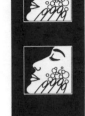

Beauty Diary

SENSATIONAL SKIN

CHAPTER TWELVE

Makeup Magic

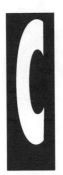

osmetics used for ritual or beautification date back to ancient times and were common in every area and culture of the world. In the Middle East, archaeologists discovered palettes used for grinding and mixing face powder as early as 6000 B.C. In Egypt, eye makeup was widely used by 4000 B.C. Egyptian women shaded their eyes with a green powder made from malachite, sometimes mixed with a glittering powder of crushed iridescent green beetle shells. The insides of their eyes were lined and their eyelashes and brows darkened with kohl, a powder made from antimony, burnt almonds, black oxide from copper, and ochre clay. Rouge was created by mixing clay with saffron, which Egyptian women applied to their cheeks.

Cosmetics were not the sole domain of Egyptian women, however, as evidenced by the generous supply of skin cream, lip color and rouge found in the tomb of King Tutankhamen. Even the Old Testament refers to face painting, indicating the Hebrews also adopted Egyptian makeup practices.

Unlike the Greeks, who favored a more natural look, Romans wholeheartedly adopted Egyptian makeup techniques, favoring the use of kohl for lining the eyes and darkening eyelashes. Although the use of cosmetics declined during the early Christian era, the Crusaders of the Middle Ages returned home with cosmetics and techniques they discovered in the East and later spread throughout Europe.

Face painting, often with poisonous artists' pigments, gained wide popularity during the Renaissance. By the 17th century, rose-colored cheek rouge, face powder and lip rouge were worn by both men and women of the upper classes. Face patches, often in the shape of stars or half-moons and worn by men and women in multiples, were first used to cover smallpox scars in the 18th century.

While makeup use became excessive in the 18th century, fashion reversed during the Victorian Age in England. Anything more than a subtle touch of powder or rouge was considered unacceptable for "nice" women. Thanks to the French, the use of cosmetics was revived. That makeup essential, mascara, was introduced by Empress Eugenie.

Unfortunately, until modern times, the composition of makeup was often toxic and deadly. The white powder, used for hundreds of years to lighten the complexion, contained large quantities of lead. Many rouges contained cinnabar, a poisonous red sulfide of mercury. Safe cosmetics were not developed and produced until the end of the 19th century in France. As a result, over-the-counter cosmetics became more widely used. Today, science and cosmetology combine to create innovative and technologically advanced cosmetics that are not only safe, but also designed for beautiful results.

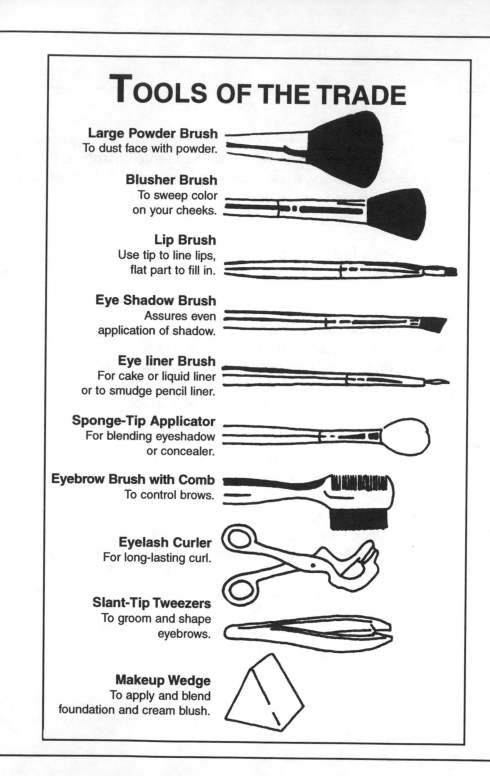

TOOLS OF THE TRADE

Large Powder Brush
To dust face with powder.

Blusher Brush
To sweep color
on your cheeks.

Lip Brush
Use tip to line lips,
flat part to fill in.

Eye Shadow Brush
Assures even
application of shadow.

Eye liner Brush
For cake or liquid liner
or to smudge pencil liner.

Sponge-Tip Applicator
For blending eyeshadow
or concealer.

Eyebrow Brush with Comb
To control brows.

Eyelash Curler
For long-lasting curl.

Slant-Tip Tweezers
To groom and shape
eyebrows.

Makeup Wedge
To apply and blend
foundation and cream blush.

901. What are the differences among liquid, stick and cake foundations and tinted moisturizer?

Stick and cake foundations provide the most coverage but are heavier and less natural looking. Liquid foundations combine sheerness and coverage. Tinted moisturizers are very sheer and provide a little color without coverage. Foundations can be oil-based or oil-free. Be sure to choose one that is compatible with your skin type.

902. How often should foundation be replaced to guard against contamination?

Foundations generally last for two to three years and do best when stored out of sunlight and in a cool location. Oil-based foundations tend to separate over time; water-based foundations tend to evaporate. Discard products whose color or texture has changed. To prevent contamination, use a disposable foundation spatula with foundations that come in a bottle or jar. Beauty Secrets offers these in packages of 12 or more.

903. How often should makeup sponges be replaced?

For better hygiene and performance, wash makeup sponges after each use in mild soapy water. Rinse well and air dry throughly. Replace when they begin to lose shape and resilience or smell moldy. Many makeup artists use Beauty Secrets wedges available in economical 100-count packages.

904. What goes on first, concealer or foundation?

Choose a concealer that closely matches your skin tone and apply it by dotting on trouble spots before your foundation. Blend well.

905. What should I use to apply foundation? How should it be applied?

For a professional look, use a firm wedge-shaped sponge. Begin by applying a small amount of foundation to the center area of your face, then blend outward toward the hairline. Blend so that the foundation disappears at the hairline and under the chin. When possible, apply foundation in natural light.

906. My skin is dry. Should I use a moisturizer under my foundation?

Yes. People with dry, normal, combination and even oily skin should always use moisturizer for their skin type under foundation. Moisturizers not only keep skin soft and smooth, but also help foundation blend easier and adhere to the skin. Try Jheri Redding Milk'N Honee moisturizers in normal-to-oily or dry-to-sensitive formulations.

907. How can I avoid a foundation line between my face and neck?

To avoid creating a makeup "mask," be sure to choose a color that closely matches your skin tone. Apply foundation in natural light and don't use more than necessary. Use a firm wedge-shaped sponge, like Beauty Secrets Makeup Wedges, to blend the line of demarcation until it disappears.

908. How can I prevent my foundation from caking?

Begin by applying a moisturizer under your foundation. Apply foundation sparingly and blend well. After a few hours, refresh your makeup with a light spritz of water from an atomizer.

909. I'm in my 20s. Do I need to use foundation for a "finished" look?

TIP   **Blend! Blend! Blend!**

Modern women wear makeup to enhance their appearance. Properly applied, daytime makeup should be subtle—never obvious—and should accentuate our good features while minimizing others. The key is to choose makeup colors that match or complement your skin tone. Apply makeup in the light in which it will be seen (bright, natural light for day; bright, incandescent for evening). Always use proper tools and remember to blend, blend, blend, using your finger tips or professional makeup sponges. When applying foundation, blend until it fades at the hairline and under the chin. When applying blush or eyeshadows, blend until there is no obvious difference between colors or tones. Evening makeup also requires subtle blending to avoid a "made-up" look. Always use professional makeup applicators—brushes and sponges. Experiment and practice to sharpen your skills.

A foundation is recommended even if your skin is young and flawless, because a minimal amount of a sheer liquid foundation evens out skin color to give your complexion extra polish. For an everyday alternative, try a dual-finish pressed powder.

910. What can I use to cover "age spots"?

To cover dark areas, or "age spots," on the skin, dab a little concealer on the area. Then apply foundation as usual, blending with a wedge-shaped sponge. Use the new, flocked makeup sponges by Beauty Secrets designed specifically for applying liquid foundation.

911. What causes those large brown spots on my face, and how can I get rid of them?

Flat "age spots" or "liver spots" can range in size from one-quarter inch to several inches and result from cumulative sun damage. Lemon juice applied to the spot is the age-old treatment and can be effective, but the acid in the juice can also cause irritation. Today, dermatologists have both surgical and chemical methods for removing lentigines, as they are medically called, but they may also be treated with over-the-counter skin bleaches. If you are acne prone, avoid greasy "fade" cream formulas.

912. Foundation and powder tend to accentuate my wrinkles, how can I avoid this?

Try using a moisturizer containing alpha hydroxy acids, like Purist Skin Therapy Day

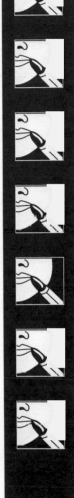

Moisture Cream, which helps to slough off dead skin cells to reveal fresher looking skin. Next, use a moisturizing foundation, blending well with a wedge-shaped sponge. Finish with a light dusting of powder. Apply powder sparingly using a professional powder brush and blend, blend, blend. Later in the day, touch-up and blend makeup with your wedge-shaped sponge.

913. My skin is oily and prone to blemishes. I need coverage but foundation tends to aggravate my skin. What can I do?

Look for an oil-free, noncomedegenic (non clogging) makeup specially formulated for oily skin. Read package labels carefully.

914. I use an oil-free foundation in the morning, but by noon my skin looks shiny. What can I do?

Try using powder blotting papers which will absorb excess oil and shine without removing your makeup. Then go over your face with pressed powder. Be sure to wash sponge or velour applicator frequently.

915. As an African-American, how can I avoid the ashen look foundations often produce?

An ashen look is produced when the foundation doesn't have enough yellow or red undertones. For best results, choose a foundation from a line specifically designed for women of color.

916. What is the difference between stage makeup and the makeup I buy at the department or drug store?

Stage makeup is often heavier and provides more coverage. It is designed to withstand harsh stage or studio lighting. Foundations purchased at the department or drug store are usually lighter and available in a wider range of shades. They tend to look more natural under normal lighting conditions.

917. When I buy foundation and powder, the colors that appear to match my skin in the store look too pink when I put them on my skin! What should I do?

In their desire for rosy-looking skin, many women choose a color with too much red in it for their natural skin tone. When choosing facial makeup, go toward more yellow-based colors. The store's artificial lighting could also be the culprit. Since makeup cannot be exchanged, check your makeup colors in natural light before purchasing.

918. Do pressed powder and loose powder produce different effects?

Yes. Loose powder (tinted or translucent) "sets" makeup and minimizes shine, but doesn't add coverage. Loose powder should be applied sparingly with a large professional powder brush, such as Body Trends Super

---

F.Y. 👁 Why Use Professional Makeup Brushes?

For model-quality makeup, use the right tools. Professional makeup brushes are designed for the demanding standards of makeup artists who know the quality of brushes, as well as the shape, affect the outcome.

Professional makeup brushes vary in size and shape. Each is designed to perform a certain task, such as line the eyes or blend powder blush. The hairs are hand-set and crimped to the handle for better shape and longer wear. The best natural hair brushes are made of sable. Mink, weasel, otter, squirrel, pony and goat hair are also used. Synthetic—nylon or nylon/poly—brushes hold creams and oils better because they are non-porous and don't absorb color and oil as natural hair does.

Some newer nylon blends are extremely soft and perform as well as or better than natural hair.

To keep brushes clean, wipe off excess makeup after every use. Store brushes away from dust and heat. Once a week, natural hair brushes can be dipped in a professional brush cleaner solution, like Beauty Secrets Brush Cleaner. Wipe with a paper towel and lay flat to air dry. Once a month, they can be washed with mild soap and water. Never dry brushes with the hair end up as water will gather inside the handle and cause damage to the brush.

Duster Brush or Powder Application Brush. Blot excess with a large puff, such as Voyez Velour Puffs. Pressed powder is denser than loose powder. It provides light coverage and may be used to refresh makeup or even in place of foundation for quick application. Use a clean velour puff or sponge to apply pressed powder.

919. What is translucent powder? How is it used and applied?

Translucent powder is used over foundation to "set" makeup, not to cover or add color. Apply translucent powder with large professional powder brush and pat with a large velour puff, like Voyez Big Blush Puff.

920. What is the difference between a dual-finish powder and pressed powder?

Pressed powder contains only powder, while dual-finish powder is foundation and powder in one product. Dual-finish powder provides more coverage than pressed powder and can be applied with a puff or with a damp makeup sponge.

921. Do I need to use powder if I use foundation?

Yes. Loose powder "sets" your foundation and helps keep it in place so it doesn't collect in your skin's creases. It gives your makeup a professional, "finished" look and reduces shine.

922. How can I select the right pressed powder color for me?

Look for a color that closely matches your skin tone in natural light. Because skin tone is not uniform, test powder on several areas of your face.

923. Can I use pressed powder instead of foundation?

Yes. You can use pressed powder instead of foundation for light coverage and quick application, but it won't provide as much coverage as foundation unless you use a dual-finish powder, also called a "wet/dry" powder. Used wet it becomes a foundation. Used dry it acts like a pressed powder.

924. Do powder, cream and liquid blushes produce different effects?

Yes. Powder blushes are easiest to apply and provide a matte finish. Cream-based blushes have more texture and provide a dewier look. Cream blushes are a good solution for older or dryer skin types. Liquid blushes have the least texture and are difficult to blend. For this reason, liquid blush is not recommended for most women.

925. I have a thin scar on my chin from an old childhood injury. What is the best way to camouflage it?

There is little you can do cosmetically to downplay the texture of a scar. Apply foundation lightly and evenly over your face. If the scar is red, try adding a little concealer and blend well. Finish by gently pressing the translucent powder with a large velour puff. Sometimes trying to camouflage a scar with heavy coverage only draws more attention to it. The best bet is to draw attention away from a scar by emphasizing your best facial features.

926. Is the brush that comes with my powder blusher adequate or should I use a special brush?

Professional makeup artists agree that the size and quality of brushes that come with most powder blushers are inadequate. You'll get superior results with professional blusher brushes, like Body Trends Deluxe Blusher Brush. Because they are larger and made of superior fiber, they blend better.

927. What's the best way to apply a cream blush?

Cream blush products should be applied with a wedge-shaped cosmetic sponge or with the finger tips. Dab a small amount on the cheekbone and blend well.

928. Where on my cheeks should I apply blush? On the cheekbone or under it?

Blush should be applied on the cheekbone where the sun would give your cheeks a rosy glow.

929. How can I use blush to create facial contours?

To create the illusion of contour, use your regular blush color on your cheekbone and apply a slightly deeper shade just underneath the cheekbone to contour. The trick is to be subtle. Don't apply too much color, and blend well.

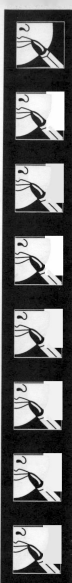

930. What are bronzing powders? How should they be used and applied?

Bronzing powders are earth-toned powders that simulate the look of being "sun-kissed" and work well on a wide variety of skin tones. Bronzing powders should be lightly dusted over the cheek bones, the bridge of the nose, above the brows and on the chin. They sometimes come with a feathery applicator and may be applied with a professional blush brush.

931. How can I prevent my makeup from turning orange?

If your makeup looks orange when you apply it, you may have chosen a color that is too warm for your skin tone. Look for a shade with pinker, cooler undertones. If your makeup looks orange because it is old and has discolored, discard it immediately. All makeup should be kept in a cool area away from direct sunlight.

932. I'm going to be married. Are there any special makeup tips for my wedding day?

Keep your makeup clean and classic. Since white garments tend to intensify makeup, give yourself a trial run a few weeks before your wedding while wearing white. If you're doing this yourself, try an enhanced version of your normal makeup. Adjust your makeup to the type of light you'll be in. You can wear more dramatic makeup for an indoor or evening wedding than a daytime or outdoor wedding. Don't forget to set your makeup with a light dusting of translucent loose powder for a smooth, long-lasting finish. For long-wear lip-

stick, use a lip liner and two coats of lipstick, blotting between coats. To seal lipstick, use lip sealer. Just brush it on and it will set your lipstick, or lightly dust transculent powder over your lips, then blot. For smudge-free eyes, be sure to use waterproof mascara. Good choices: Beautique Lip Liners, Beauty Selectives Lip Savvy Professional Formula Lip Color with matching nail enamel and Sherani Professional Water Proof Mascara provide excellent quality and super value.

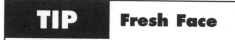

TIP   Fresh Face

To help keep makeup fresh and free of bacteria, always wash hands before touching makeup products. Keep containers tightly closed and store in a cool, dry place. Keep a purse-sized hand sanitizer like Beauty Secrets Gel Sanitizer with you for touch-ups on the go.

933. What is the best way to remove makeup thoroughly?

Water-based makeup can be removed with mild soap and water. Oil-based and water-proof makeup require a specially formulated makeup remover. Use quilted cotton pads such as Beauty Secrets 100% cotton rounds or squares or Beauty Secrets Professional Red Make-up Sponges. Avoid cotton balls and tissues because their loose fibers can cause irritation.

934. How should I adjust my makeup in the summer when my skin tans?

When skin is lightly tanned, you'll need to use warmer colors than your winter indoor

palette. Try using a tinted moisturizer instead of foundation and more deeply or richly toned lipsticks. Limit your sun exposure to achieve just a healthy glow and always apply sunscreen. Remember, the sun that tans your skin also damages it, causing premature aging and even skin cancer.

935. My foundation has an SPF of 15. Is it necessary to also wear a sunscreen under my foundation if I will be going out in the sun?

If your makeup has an SPF of 15, it is not necessary to wear a separate sunscreen product under your foundation. However, remember that to achieve adequate coverage you must apply the foundation over all exposed areas. Keep in mind that perspiration or swimming will wash away the makeup and the protection.

936. How can I quickly and easily change my makeup to take me from day to evening?

The easiest way to create an evening look is to intensify your day look. Try a darker or richer color lipstick, lining your lips first with a matching pencil liner. Add eye liner, deepen your eye shadow, refresh your mascara and re-groom your eyebrows. Brush on a little blush, and off you go.

937. My makeup looks great indoors, but sometimes looks too harsh outside. What can I do?

Makeup can look completely different exposed to different levels and types of light. Try to apply your makeup in the brightest light it will be exposed to. Best bet is to apply makeup in bright, natural light, facing a window so that the light reflects on your face.

938. Should I use a lighted makeup mirror?

The light you use when making up should be as close as possible to the light in which you are going to be seen. There are many mirrors on the market with bulbs that simulate various lighting conditions. It's not necessary to use a lighted makeup mirror. Bright, natural light is always best for daytime makeup.

939. In what order should I apply my eye liner, eye shadow and mascara?

Apply eye shadow first, then liner, and finally mascara. Shadow goes on first so that it does not obscure the eye liner, which requires the least amount of blending. Mascara goes on last to prevent smudging.

940. What should I use to apply eye shadow, a brush or a sponge applicator?

Eye shadows with heavy pigment should be applied with a professional eye shadow brush to blend strong color well. Eye shadows with less pigment should be applied with a disposable sponge applicator which applies more product. To test whether your eye shadow has a lot of pigment, touch it lightly with a clean finger tip. If your finger tip shows a lot of color, the product contains heavy pigment. Try Beauty Secrets Sponge Tip Applicators or Casaro Double Tip Make-up Applicators.

941. My eye shadow seems to disappear during the day. How can I make it last longer?

Use an under-eye concealer or base on lids. You can also switch to an eye shadow with more pigment or reapply your shadow as needed. Pencils last longer than powders because of their waxy consistency.

942. My eye shadow gathers in the crease of my eye. What can I do to prevent this?

Eye shadow tends to slide on your skin's oil. To prevent this, first dust your eyelid with translucent powder, then apply your eye shadow with a professional shadow brush or sponge tipped applicator.

943. What is the best way to apply eye liner, with a brush or a pencil?

Brushes and pencils produce different eye liner looks. Eye liner applied with a professional eye liner brush will produce a finer, more intense line for a more dramatic look. Pencils produce a thicker line and are better for smudging or blending. Because applying a fine line with a brush requires some skill, many people find pencils more user friendly.

944. How can I achieve a defined, long-lasting line with my eye liner?

For a clean line, use a water-based, cake eye liner, a professional eye liner brush, a good magnifying mirror and a steady hand. Cake eye liners are easier for amateurs than water-proof liquid liners because mistakes can be erased.

945. What are eyelash curlers? How are they used?

Eyelash curlers are mechanical devices that bend the eyelashes, causing your eyes to appear larger and your lashes longer. Use an eyelash curler before you apply mascara. There are several different eyelash curlers on the market. One of the best is the Tweezerman Eyelash Curler with a no-stick rubber pad you can warm with a blow dryer for a longer lasting curl. To use, press lashes gently with the curler. For a natural look, repeat three times, each time moving away from the lash line.

946. Since I have started curling my eyelashes my eyelids have become red and swollen. Could my eyelash curler be a problem?

You could be allergic to the nickel plating on your eyelash curler, or to the chemical MBT used to preserve the rubber coating on the curler ends. Consult a dermatologist to confirm the source of the problem.

947. How often should I replace my eyelash curler?

Replace your eyelash curler when it loses its tension or when you notice build-up like rust or corrosion. You can wash your eyelash curler after each use, but be sure to dry thoroughly.

948. Help! Every time I wear mascara, I end up with raccoon eyes. What am I doing wrong?

The primary solution to this problem is to avoid touching your eyes. All mascara will smudge if you touch or rub your eyes. Try a waterproof or non-smudge professional formula mascara, like Sherani Waterproof Mascara.

949. When I apply mascara, it clumps. What can I do?

This problem could be partially due to the type of mascara you are using. Mascara termed "lash thickeners" or "lash builders" tend to be thicker and may clump more easily. There are two solutions to this problem. Either try a mascara with a thinner formulation for a more natural look, or use a metal-tooth lash comb from Tweezerman to remove the clumps and separate lashes. You may simply need to replace your mascara. Professional makeup artists use disposable mascara applicators, like those made by Beauty Secrets.

950. Is there a special technique for applying mascara to make my lashes look thicker?

A light dusting of translucent powder before you apply your mascara will thicken your lashes. Then, apply a second coat of mascara.

951. My eyelashes are blonde, but I hate wearing mascara. Is it safe to have them tinted?

Yes. It is safe to have your eyelashes tinted, but eyelash tinting should only be done in a salon by a skilled professional with the correct products. Some dye formulas are dangerous to use in the eye area. Many fair-haired women find eyelash tinting a convenient and carefree beauty solution.

952. How long does eyelash tinting last?

Eyelash tinting generally lasts between two and four weeks.

953. I love the look of false eyelashes for special occasions. How do I choose and apply them?

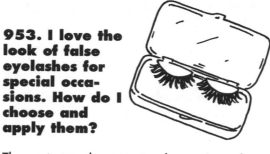

The easiest and most natural way to apply false eyelashes is to use individual lashes with a medium flare. Squeeze a tiny drop of Ardell Lashtite Adhesive—glue specially formulated for applying false eyelashes—on your finger and dip the tip of the lash into glue. Insert individual lashes between your natural lashes spacing them a little less than 1/4" apart, starting at the outer corner of your eye and working inward. Ardell's Duralash eyelashes come in short, medium or long, and in black or brown.

954. Should I apply eye makeup before or after false eyelashes?

Before putting on false eyelashes, apply all your other makeup. Then apply the false eyelashes. Finish with mascara (if necessary).

955. What is the best way to remove false eyelashes?

Remove false eyelashes by gently pulling them off your eyelid. Follow up with eye makeup remover pads to remove the excess lash adhesive. Individual lashes should be removed with Lash Free Adhesive Remover or mineral oil.

956. My eyebrows are wild. How can I tame them?

For well-groomed brows, use an eyebrow brush like Body Trends Lash/Brow Groomer to shape and control. For very unruly brows, brush with a tiny dab of hair gel or mustache wax, like Clubman's.

957. My eyebrows need shaping. Are there any guidelines?

Nature provides each of us with the right brow shape. While brows often need grooming, it's best not to radically alter the natural contour of your brows. Use professional slant-tip tweezers, such as those by Tweezerman, to clean up the area between brows and to pluck stray hairs underneath brows to create an arch. Never tweeze above the brows—you'll alter the natural shape. Brows should start just above the inner corner of the eye and extend slightly past the outer corner of the eye. To get the endpoints of your brows right, try this professional trick: First, hold a pencil vertically, point end up, in front of the center of the eye. Next, tip the pencil until the eraser hits the side of your nose and note where the point end meets your eyebrow. This is where your brow should end on the outside. Now hold the pencil vertically, placing it next to your nose. Note where the pencil meets the eyebrow. This is where your brow should start on the inside. Brows may also be waxed by a professional esthetician. Don't try it yourself, though!

958. Is it true that over-plucked brows won't grow back?

No. The only way to keep hair from growing back is to destroy the hair root (papilla), which is usually done by electrolysis. It can take plucked hairs up to eight weeks to grow back.

959. How can I best fill in sparse areas in my eyebrows?

Fill eyebrow in with an eyebrow pencil, using light strokes. You can also try using an eye shadow in a shade that matches your natural hair color, applying it with a stiff, wedge-shaped brush.

960. Is there a special technique to using an eyebrow pencil?

Light strokes give a more natural look. You can also blend the pencil with a stiff brush.

961. I color my hair. Can I color my eyebrows too?

Yes. Eyebrows can easily be colored when you color your hair. However, because proper formula and technique are essential, this is a procedure that should be done by a professional.

962. How can I enhance my eyes and still have a soft, natural look?

Try using eye shadow instead of eye liner. Take a dark color and blend it close to the lash line. Then apply a coat of a "natural-look" mascara.

963. How can I achieve the "smoky" eyes I see in magazines?

Use a dark, intense eye shadow color and blend it very well with a professional eye shadow brush, all the way around the eye, from corner to corner, on brow bone and eyelid. Blending is essential for a "smoky" look.

964. How can I get that "nude" look I see on high-fashion models?

The easiest way to create a "no makeup" look with polish is to choose eye shadow shades in soft beige, brown and vanilla tones. Apply foundation to entire eye area, then brush lids with a slightly deeper tone, using an even deeper shade in the crease. Apply vanilla-tone shadow under brow. Blend, blend, blend. Finish with brown or clear mascara.

965. I'm getting married. Are there special eye makeup tips for wedding photos?

Keep your makeup simple and classic to give your wedding photos a timeless quality. Apply your makeup in natural light and keep in mind that makeup appears more intense when you wear white. Avoid frosted or metallic eye shadows because the iridescent particles tend to gather and accentuate fine lines. Use waterproof mascara, but avoid heavy

false eyelashes which often cast dark shadows under the eyes. Don't apply any new makeup products without a trial run to test for both allergic reaction and color correctness.

966. I have dark circles under my eyes, but when I apply concealer, they look too light! How can I achieve the right balance?

Try choosing a concealer in a slightly darker shade. Don't use a concealer that is lighter than your own skin tone. Instead, choose your concealer to match your skin tone and keep in mind that it is natural to have light shadows under the contour of your eyes. Dark circles benefit from a yellow-based concealer. Dot concealer over dark circles.

967. My eyes are so small. How can I make them appear larger?

Avoid lining your eyes. While lining defines the eyes, it also tends to close them. The solution to this problem is to create the illusion that the entire eye area is larger by gently shading the entire eyelid. Shaping the arch of the eyebrows and applying a highlighter under the brow can also open up eyes.

968. My eyes are spaced too closely together. How can I make them look more wide-set?

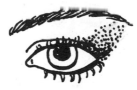

Apply a light-colored eye shadow or concealer to the inner corner of the eye and blend well. Accentuate the outer corners using eye liner, shadow and mascara.

showing colors that seem
to change in different lights

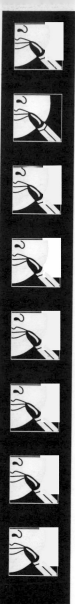

969. My eyes are too widely set. How can I make them appear more closely spaced?

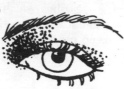

Wide-set eyes are often due to a wider nose bridge. The solution here is to shade the inside corner of the eye and along the inside bridge of the nose with a neutral-tone eye shadow, blending well with a professional eye shadow brush or sponge.

970. My eyes are deep-set. How can I bring them out?

Avoid using dark eye shadows and don't use shadow in the crease of your eyelid. To bring your eyes out, try using a light-color eye shadow on your eyelid.

971. My eyes protrude. How can I make them appear to recede?

To set your eyes back, use a dark shadow on your eyelid. If your eyes are large or round, apply an eye liner first.

972. I have blue eyes and fair skin. What eye shadow shades are best for me?

For the most natural look, use shades of pink/beige and brown on your lid and in the crease. For a more dramatic look, try gray tones. For a more colorful look, try subtle shades of slate, mauve and violet.

973. I have deep, dark brown eyes and chestnut brown hair. What are my best eye shadow shades?

For deep brown eyes and chestnut brown hair, try a warm, light, neutral beige tone on the lid, and a darker brown for the crease of your eye. For more drama, use shades of charcoal and black.

TIP   **Clear Colors**

If you love the color but hate the intensity, tone down your bright-colored lipsticks. Apply an even coat of color—a lipstick brush works best—and top it with a clear gloss. The result is still vibrant but less intense.

---

974. I am an African-American woman with very dark skin. What eye shadow colors should I select and what should I avoid?

Avoid iridescents and pale pastels that will look ashy on your skin. For very dark skin, use a deep brown or black shadow. For more color, use plum, prune or other deeply saturated colors.

975. I have hazel eyes and auburn hair. What are the most flattering eye shadow colors for me?

For a natural look, try warm browns, banana or apricot. For more drama, try greens, khaki, red/brown or gold.

976. I wear contact lenses. What type of eye makeup is right for me?

Avoid iridescent shadows because they may contain mica or other irritants. If possible, put your contacts in after you apply your eye makeup. A 4X mirror may be helpful, such as Voyez Magic Eye Flex Stand or Double 4X Compact Mirror.

977. Should I use more eye makeup if I wear glasses?

Eyes do look different behind lenses. If you're nearsighted, your eyes will appear to recede behind your lenses. Use a light neutral shadow on your eyelid and brow bone. Contour with a slightly darker shade in the crease. Line your top lid only and apply mascara. If you're farsighted, your lenses will magnify your eyes. Use a medium neutral shadow on your eyelids with a slightly darker shade in the crease. Avoid bright or shiny colors.

978. Can I really swim with waterproof eye makeup?

Yes. However, keep in mind that cool water, particularly, may cause your mascara to flake. Also, keep in mind that after swimming, wet lashes may feel heavy. To dry wet eyes, pat gently. Avoid the impulse to wipe your eyes after swimming as wiping will smear your makeup.

979. Should I use a magnifying mirror when I put on eye makeup?

Use a magnifying mirror if it makes applying eye makeup easier for you. A magnifying mirror may be especially helpful to contact lens wearers who prefer to apply their makeup before putting in their lenses. Remember, with or without a magnifying mirror, it's always best to apply makeup in natural light. Daylight complements skin tone and reveals the full color spectrum.

980. I've often heard that eye makeup should be replaced frequently to guard against contamination. What are the guidelines?

Because bacteria spread more easily in liquid makeup products than powder, mascara is the most perishable eye makeup and should be replaced every three months. Try not to touch the wand to anything but your eyelashes. Keep the case tightly closed and store in a cool place. Don't use mascara if the smell or texture has changed. Pencil eye liner lasts for up to three years. Sharpening with a clean, professional sharpener decreases the chance of contamination. Powder eye shadows should last for three years or longer but can become flaky with age. Clean eye makeup brushes and wash sponge applicators weekly with a mild soap and water. Replace as necessary. To extend the life of your cosmetics, consider using disposable cosmetic spatulas and mascara wands available from Beauty Secrets.

981. I have just had an eye lift and want to start wearing eye makeup again. When is it safe to wear my makeup again?

Consult your physician before you begin to wear makeup again. Because eye makeup is most susceptible to bacteria contamination, it is advisable to use new makeup and applicators after surgical procedures.

982. When applying my eye makeup, I invariably end up with smudges where I don't want them. What is a quick and easy way to erase smudges without having to start over?

Dip a cotton swab in eye makeup remover, and gently wipe the area. Blot with translucent powder.

983. What is the difference between lipstick, lip stain and lip gloss?

Lipsticks have both texture (matte, cream, glossy, frosted) and color (pigment). Lip stains give a hint of color without a high shine. Glosses impart lots of shine and translucent color.

TIP | **Well Protected**

Foundation containing sunscreen can protect your skin from damaging ultraviolet rays, but be sure to check the SPF factor. If the SPF is below 15, dermatologists recommend using a separate sunscreen under your foundation.

---

984. Why do makeup pros use a lip brush to apply lipstick?

A professional lip brush gives a more precise line and coverage than lipstick in a tube. Body Trends Retractable Lip Brush or Beauty Secrets Disposable Lipstick Brushes are great for popping in your purse or makeup drawer at home.

985. How can I define the shape of my lips?

Define the outline of your lips with a professional lip brush or a lip liner pencil that closely matches the color of your lipstick. Then apply your lipstick with the lip brush, blending the liner with the brush.

986. My lipstick disappears so fast. How can I make it last longer?

A matte formulation with more pigment (color) and less emollients (oils) lasts longer. These lipsticks are usually labeled "long-lasting." Glosses, lip shines or stain formulations contain less pigment and wear off more quickly. Layering also helps lipstick last longer. Apply lipstick with a professional lip brush, blot with a tissue, then reapply. Makeup artists often use lip liner as a foundation. Choose a lip liner pencil that is the same color as your lipstick, outline your lips and then fill in all over with the pencil. Apply lipstick with a professional lipstick brush over the lip liner base. Try Beauty Selectives Professional Lip Savvy Lip Color. There are several lipsticks, Brucci Changes or Jade Lipstick, available with an aloe vera base that apply clear and then change to a rose, red or coral tone, depending on your body chemistry. These are particularly effective when used as a base for your lipstick.

987. How do I keep lipstick on all day?

Try a lipstick sealer, like Claudia Stevens Lipstick Sealer, over lipstick, or apply a lip base, like Brucci Changes Lipstick, before

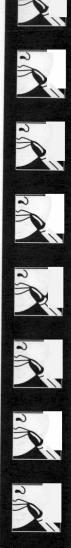

using lipstick. Apply lipstick, blot, then apply again. Do not blot final coat. Using a lip liner as lipstick also works well!

988. Should lipstick be blotted? I've heard conflicting advice.

Blotting removes some of the lipstick from your lips, giving more of a stained look that some women prefer. Blotting, then re-applying lipstick helps lipstick last longer on lips.

989. How can I keep my lipstick from bleeding?

Using a lip liner pencil first helps prevent bleeding because the waxy ingredients in the pencil create a barrier.

990. Are lip liners the only thing available to prevent lipstick from bleeding?

No. You can also try a lip sealer. Lip sealers are products you apply over lipstick to seal it. Another suggestion is to select a matte lipstick formulation which is dryer and contains more pigment. Lip glosses, lip shines or cream formulations contain less pigment and the emollients they contain tend to bleed more. Try Claudia Stevens Lipstick Sealer and Claudia Stevens Anti-Feathering Lip Base or Young Lips Lip Wrinkle Cream.

991. My lips are thin. How can I make them appear fuller?

To create the illusion of fullness, start by using a pencil lip liner to define the outermost part of your lip line. Apply your lipstick with a pro-

fessional lip brush, blending the lip liner, and add a slightly lighter color in the center to create contour. Avoid dark-colored lipsticks.

992. My lips are very full. How can I minimize them?

Full lips are often considered sensual and beautiful. But if you want to minimize full lips, use a lip liner pencil, like Beautique's professional lip liner pencils, to define the inside of your natural lip line. Fill in with lipstick or Beautique's Lip Crayon. Try a slightly deeper colored lipstick.

TIP   **Soft Sculpture**

To create soft facial contours, apply a very small amount of contour powder, starting at the ear and sweeping toward the middle of the face. Blend well with a large brush. Apply a small amount of blush just above the contour. Blend again. Go slowly, using products sparingly and working in bright light. Step back and take a look; if the effect is obvious, you've used too much.

---

993. In cold weather my lips become dry and chapped. Should I apply a lip balm or moisturizer under my lipstick?

The emollients in moisturizers and lip balms could interfere with the adherence of your lipstick, so try using a moisturizing lipstick instead. To help cold-nipped lips, apply petroleum jelly or aloe-based lip balm, such as At

One Lip Moisturizing Treatment or Beyond Belief Lip Balm, at night before bed.

994. I love the look of matte lipsticks, but they make my lips too dry. What can I do?

For a non-drying, matte look, try applying a cream formulation and blotting it with a tissue. Repeat for longer lasting coverage.

995. My skin is sun sensitive. Do lipsticks with sunscreen provide enough protection?

Sun-sensitive lips need protection at the SPF 15 level. Check the label to make sure the lipstick you're interested in is rated with SPF 15.

996. I love outdoor sports but hate the look of white sunblocks. Is there a more attractive alternative for my sun-sensitive lips?

You can wear a lip balm, like Beyond Belief Lip Balm with SPF 15, a salve or even lipstick, as long as it has maximum sun protection. Look for SPF 15 or higher on the package.

997. After 40 years of wearing the same lipstick, I have developed an allergy to it, causing my lips to burn, swell and sometimes result in fever blisters. What ingredient could be causing my allergy? Should I use a hypoallergenic lipstick?

After 40 years, the manufacturer may have changed the formula and added a product that you are sensitive to. Also, over time your tolerance for certain ingredients may have diminished. Try changing the shade and then the brand of lipstick you are currently using. Hypo-allergenic products contain fewer allergy-causing ingredients than other products and are usually fragrance-free.

998. I'm going to be married. Are there any special lipstick tips for wedding photos?

Be sure to use a lip liner pencil to give your lips good definition. Avoid using a very glossy lipstick; it may cause unwanted highlights, and won't last as long as a matte lipstick. Consider using a lip sealer, like Claudia Stevens Lipstick Sealer.

999. I am Asian and want to choose the correct makeup colors for my complexion. What guidelines should I consider?

Choose foundation in beige tones from ivory to medium. Avoid pink tones. Use shading or contouring powder instead of blusher. For more cheek color, choose apricot or rose powder blusher on cheekbones. Use gray or brown pencil eye liners to emphasize the natural shape of eyes. If skin tone is light, avoid pink lip color, choosing light, clear reds, cranberry and soft coral lip shades. If skin is dark, pale pinks or corals are good options.

1000. Does "unscented" and "fragrance-free" on my cosmetics mean the same thing?

While the terms "unscented" and "fragrance-free" are used somewhat interchangeably, they are not precisely the same. "Unscented" generally means that the manufacturer has not added a specific fragrance to the product. "Fragrance-free" implies that the product has no odor. However, even if the product has no scent or odor, it may contain masking fragrances that serve to block the odor of other ingredients. Fragrance is the most common cause of allergic skin reactions to cosmetics.

1001. I recently had cosmetic surgery to re-shape my nose. When can I begin to wear regular makeup again?

There is no universal answer to this question. Be sure to consult your doctor before resuming your normal makeup routine. When you do begin, be especially careful to keep all applicators clean and bacteria-free.

TIP **Just BROWSing**

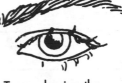

To make eyebrows appear thinner, apply color in the center of each brow. For a heavier look, apply color throughout the brow. To emphasize the brow's natural shape, work pencil at the top of the brow, brushing brows up and keeping them in place with a brow gel, colorless mascara or even mustache wax!

Beauty Diary

MAKEUP MAGIC

Glossary

ABS Plastic:
The substance from which most artificial nail tips are made.

Accelerator (related to the nails):
Applied to the nails in between layers of wrap application to help glue dry faster.

Acetone:
The main ingredient in nail polish removers for natural nails.

Acid Perm:
A permanent wave product with a pH from 6.5 to 8.0. Generally, acid waves are milder products, producing soft, loose, natural-looking curls.

Acne:
A disorder of the skin caused by inflammation of the skin glands and hair follicles.

Acrylic:
The material out of which sculptured nails are created. Acrylic is made by combining a liquid and a powder which, when applied onto nails and allowed to dry and harden, forms a tough, artificial surface.

Activator:
An ingredient added to bleach which increases the speed of bleaching action without harming the hair. Activators are known by several names, including Bleach Boosters or Accelerators.

Alkaline Perm:
A permanent wave product with a pH from 7.5 to 9.5. Generally, alkaline waves are stronger, producing firm, crisp, springy curls.

Alpha Hydroxy Acid:
A group of several naturally occurring acids that lift dead skin cells from the underlying skin, making skin appear clearer and more even-toned. AHAs are present in a broad spectrum of skin care products.

Ammonia:
A strong, alkaline substance found in some (but not all) permanent hair color. Ammonia sends a chemical signal to the developer, to lighten (decolorize) the hair.

Ammonium Thioglycolate:
The active chemical ingredient in permanent waves and ethnic curl products. Nicknamed "thio" in the beauty industry.

Antioxidants:
A substance that opposes oxidation or inhibits reactions promoted by oxygen or peroxide.

Aromatherapy:
Therapeutic use of botanical essences.

Ash:
The term used by many manufacturers for a "cool," green-based hair color.

Astringent:
Solution that helps remove oil from skin.

Barbicide:
The brand name of a sanitizing solution commonly used to sterilize salon implements.

Base Cream:
A protective cream that is applied to the forehead, ears and neck before relaxing (or curling) to minimize skin contact with chemicals.

Basecoat:
A clear, thick polish applied before nail color to provide a smooth surface and help the other coats of polish adhere better.

Benzoyl Peroxide:
An effective anti-acne medication that works by both killing acne-provoking bacteria in the follicles and slightly discouraging oil gland production.

Bisulfate Perm:
A perm that has bisulfate, a chemical compound that can curl hair.

Blackheads:
A mixture of dead skin cells, oil and bacteria.

Bleach(ing):
To chemically strip some color from the hair. Also referred to as decolorizing or pre-lightening.

Bleeding (Lipstick):
When lipstick runs off the outline of lips, creating a streaked look.

Blotting:
To remove some lipstick from lips by using tissue.

Boar Bristle:
Bristle comes from the wild boar, usually found in India or China.

Body Wave:
Another term for a permanent wave or an ethnic curl product.

Body:
The quality of liveliness or springiness of hair

Bonding:
A temporary way to add more hair to a person's head. Locks of synthetic or human hair are attached to existing hair strands with glue.

Botanical:
Containing plants, or ingredients made from plants.

Brassy:
The term for unflattering yellow, red or orange tones in some hair colors. Hair can turn "brassy" from overexposure to sun, wind or chemicals, or from lightening the hair.

Bronzers:
Powders that are brushed on like blush which contain water soluble pigment to make skin appear darker.

Buffer (related to nails):
An extremely fine-grit file used for shining the surface of the nail.

Buffer (related to skin):
A thick, protective cream which can be applied to the face and skin during a color process to prevent stains.

Calluses:
Dry patches of dead, hardened skin.

Cetyl Alcohol:
An ingredient in some conditioners and styling aids, which smoothes and softens hair.

Chelating:
A deep-cleansing process, also known as "clarifying," to lightly strip the hair before a chemical service.

Citric Acid:
A common ingredient in post-perm treatment products, which gives hair a fresh scent and helps eliminate perm odor.

Clarifying Shampoo:
A type of shampoo designed for deep-cleansing, to remove something from the hair: chlorine, hard water minerals or a build-up of styling aids. Clarifying shampoos have a slightly higher (more alkaline) pH than everyday shampoo

Cleansing Creams:
Oil-based moisturizers used mainly for cleansing purposes, although they contain little or no soap or detergent. Meant to be applied and wiped off, rather than washed off with water.

Cold Wave:
Another term for a permanent wave or an ethnic curl product.

Color Filler:
A substance which can be applied during the hair coloring process to ensure more uniform, natural-looking results. A filler takes the place of missing color pigment in the hair.

Color Remover:
Used to remove artificial color from hair. Some color removers take permanent color out of hair; others will only remove semi-permanent color.

Condition(ing):
To provide moisture and nutrients to the hair. Conditioning products combat dryness and make hair easier to style.

Cool:
Refers to blue, violet or green-based tones in hair colors.

Cornrows:
Fine, tight braids.

Cortex:
The middle layer of an individual hair, which makes up about three-quarters of the hairshaft. The pigment which gives hair its color is located in this layer.

Cream Rinse:
A mixture of wax, thickeners, and a group of chemicals used to condition hair.

Crimping Iron:
A thermal styling appliance that presses a loose, wavy pattern into hair.

Crown:
The topmost part of the skull or the head.

Curl Activator (Moisturizer):
A maintenance product for chemically curled hair, used to moisturize hair, make it feel softer, and "revive" the curl.

Curl(ing):
An ethnic permanent wave.

Cuticle (related to hair):
The outer layer of the hairshaft. It is made up of multiple layers of translucent cells, which overlap each other like shingles on a roof. When the layers are smooth and flat against each other, the hair reflects more light and looks shiny.

Cuticle (related to nails):
The rim of skin that surrounds the nail and prevents dirt and bacteria from getting down under it and causing infection.

Cuticle Oil (Creme):
A treatment that is massaged into the cuticle area for nourishment and moisture.

Cuticle Stick:
A wood or metal stick used to push back excess cuticle from the nail plate.

Dandruff:
Tiny flakes of dead skin cells from the scalp. There are two kinds: oily and dry dandruff.

Deep-Penetrating Treatment:
A conditioning product for occasional use, which is more intensive than an everyday conditioner. Treatments are formulated to revive dry, brittle hair by adding protein, vitamins and moisture. Some require heat; others do not.

Depilatory:
An agent for removing hair.

Disulfide Bonds:
The strongest of hair's chemical bonds, which gives each hairshaft its shape. Relaxing breaks these bonds; curling disconnects and then re-shapes them.

Double Process:
A color service which requires two steps to complete: first, lightening the existing hair color with bleach; and second, applying new color.

Elasticity:
The hair's ability to stretch without breaking, and then return to its original shape. Elasticity determines how well the hair will "hold" a curl, a major factor in choosing the correct type of perm.

Electrolysis:
The destruction of hair roots with an electric current.

Emollients:
Ingredients that soften or soothe.

Enamel:
Another term for nail polish.

End Wraps (Papers):
Small squares of paper (or other fabric) used to keep the ends of a strand of hair smooth and separated as it is rolled onto a perm rod. They're used so the hair will curl evenly along its entire length.

Exfoliating:
A process of removing dead skin cells on the top layer of skin.

Exothermic Perm:
A permanent wave product that creates its own heat chemically is "exothermic."

Extension (nail):
An artificial addition which gives length to a natural nail. Nail tips, wraps, gels and sculptured acrylic nails are all different types of nail extensions.

Extension (hair):
An artificial weft of hair, synthetic or human, used to increase the length or fullness of hair.

Fill (fill-in):
The regular service done to maintain artificial nails. Includes filing and/or adding more material at the back of the nail to blend in new growth.

"Finger" Diffuser:
Attachment to blow dryer which is used to lift and separate hair and add volume while drying hair.

Finishing Spray:
A hairspray with medium hold, which contains enough memory resins to keep a style in place for a full day.

Flat Iron:
A thermal styling appliance that straightens hair by pressing it between two flat metal plates.

Foam Foundation:
A lightweight piece of soft foam which can be cut, shaped and pinned beneath the hair to create a bun or "roll." Also called a "ratt."

Follicle:
The passageway in the scalp through which a single shaft of hair grows out.

Formaldehyde:
A chemical used in nail polishes to make them adhere better, and in strengthening treatments to penetrate and harden the nail plate.

Formaldehyde-Free:
Products which do not contain formaldehyde.

Freezing Spray:
The firmest-hold type of hairspray, good for spot styling or hard-to-hold hair.

French Manicure:
A style of nail polish application which uses two shades of polish, matched to the customer's skin tone, to make the nails look "natural" but flawless.

Frosting:
Pulling several fine strands of hair through a "frosting cap" and using bleach to remove color.

Fungus:
An infection which can grow under artificial—or even natural—nails. Nail fungus often turns the nail bed white and flaky.

Gel (related to the nails):
A type of nail hardener, overlay or nail extension which is "cured" or hardened using heat or a special UV lamp.

Grease:
A common term for hairdressings with the consistency of Vaseline.

Grit:
The texture (coarse, medium or fine) of a nail file.

Hairdressing:
A maintenance product that adds oil to hair and the scalp and gives the hair sheen. A hairdressing can also provide styling support, depending on its consistency.

Hair Shiner:
A liquid or spray applied to styled hair to mask split ends and make the hair appear instantly shinier. Most hair shiners contain silicone, which lightly coats the cuticle and "fills in" the split, damaged areas.

Hangnail:
A bit of skin hanging loose at the side or root of the fingernail.

Hardener:
Another name for a nail strengthener.

Henna:
A vegetable dye from the henna plant, which has been used since ancient times to color hair. Its dried leaves and stems are crushed into fine powder, then applied as a paste to dry hair. Traditional henna gives a reddish-orange hue.

Highlighting:
Lightening and coloring hair selectively. The technique can be done with squares of foil or other material, or a special kind of plastic "tipping cap." Small strands of hair are highlighted selectively to create a "layered" or

"sun-streaked" effect. Also known as frosting, tipping or wrapping.

Hot Comb:
A heated hair-relaxation tool.

Humectant:
An ingredient in hair products that draws moisture into the hair from the air.

Hydrogen Peroxide:
The chemical ingredient in a developer which, when mixed with permanent hair color, triggers the lifting power of the tint, and creation of molecules of new color.

Hypo-Allergenic:
Formulated to be less likely to cause an allergic reaction in sensitive people.

In-Between Type Color:
A newer type of hair color product, which combines the gentleness of semi-permanent color with the long-lasting qualities of permanent color. In-between type color requires a mild catalyst to work (peroxide).

Iron(ing):
A term for thermal straightening.

Keratin:
Both hair and nails are made up of this strong protein. Keratin contains 20 different amino acids.

Lacquer:
Another term for nail polish.

Level System:
The chart used by hair color manufacturers to identify and label hair color along two "dimensions." There are 10 levels (depths) of hair color, from Level 1 (black hair) to Level 10 (lightest blonde). There are also a half-dozen or so tones, from "warmest" red to "coolest" ash.

Level:
The depth of a hair color's shade—whether it is light, medium or dark.

Lift:
A comb that has regular teeth on one end, and a wider-toothed pick on the other.

Lift (related to hair color):
To lighten the hair color. "High-lift" means to lighten it a lot.

Lift(ing):
Separation of an artificial nail from the natural nail, or the natural nail from the nail plate.

Lip Balm:
Lip product for dry or chapped lips.

Lip Sealer:
Lip product that seals lipstick.

Lip Stain:
Lip product that gives hint of color without a high shine.

Liquid Wrap:
A type of strengthener that contains tiny fibers of a fabric to reinforce the surface of the nail.

Loofah:
A natural sponge made from a loofah plant, sometimes made into a cloth or a mitt.

Low Lights:
Using the same process as highlighting, instead of lightening hair, the stylist slightly darkens blonde hair using permanent hair color in a slightly darker shade to create a more natural look.

Lunula:
This is the "half-moon" visible on your nail.

Lye:
The common term for a relaxer product that contains sodium hydroxide as its active chemical ingredient.

Mantle:
The skin at the base of the fingernail. The mantle is directly over the matrix.

Marcel Waves:
Deep, all-over waves created by "finger wav-

ing" wet hair and allowing it to dry in the wave pattern. Wave clips typically are used to hold the waves in place as hair dries.

Matrix:
The spot, just under the skin of the mantle, where the nail plate starts growing.

Medicated Cleansers:
These contain antibacterial ingredients or topical drugs, such as benzoyl peroxide, salicylic acid, sulfur or resorcinol. Recommended for oily, acne-prone skin.

Melanin:
The pigment that makes up hair's natural color. Molecules of melanin are found in the cortex. There are two types of melanin: eumelanin is black pigment, and pheomelanin is red/yellow pigment.

Metallic Dyes:
Comb-through hair dyes which derive their color from lead or other metallic "salts." They appear to change the hair color gradually, since they build up on the hairshaft with successive applications.

Moisturize:
To add moisture; or to close the hair cuticle to prevent loss of moisture.

Mousse:
A styling foam which provides light hold, adding lift and fullness to hairstyles.

Nail Bed:
The skin beneath the nail plate.

Nail Plate:
The hard part of the natural nail that's usually called the "fingernail."

Nail Scrub:
A lightly abrasive nail cleanser used to remove yellowing and stains.

Nail Treatment:
One of a number of types of products designed to strengthen, nourish or protect the

nails. Treatments do more than simply make nails look better; they "treat" a problem, like cracking or peeling.

Neck Strip:
A sanitary strip of paper or fabric which is wrapped around a client's neck under the towel or cape during any salon services, a perm or any other chemical service.

Neutralizer:
The chemical applied at the end of a curl or relaxer service to completely stop the chemical process and return the hair to its normal pH level. A curl neutralizer is a lotion; in the relaxing process, it's usually a neutralizing shampoo.

Nippers:
Tools for trimming cuticles or nails that are more precise than scissors.

No-Base Relaxer:
A relaxer which does not require application of a base cream to the entire scalp before use.

No-Lye:
The common term for a relaxer product that contains calcium hydroxide as its active chemical ingredient. A few lye formulas contain lithium hydroxide or potassium hydroxide instead.

Non-Acetone:
Nail polish remover that contains ethyl acetate or methyl ethyl ketone as its active ingredient, instead of acetone. Recommended for use on extensions.

Noncomedegenic:
Refers to a product that will not clog the pores.

Oil Sheen:
Another term for a sheen spray.

Overprocessed:
Hair that is dry, brittle and damaged from chemical treatments.

PABA:
Para-Aminobenzoic Acid is a substance which absorbs ultraviolet light and acts as a "sun block." PABA is used in skin and hair care products, as well as tanning lotions.

Panthenol:
Vitamin B-5, which conditions and "plumps" the hairshaft to make it appear thicker.

Paraffin (Wrap):
A waxy substance used in heat treatments by manicurists and aestheticians.

Perm Rejuvenator (also called a Revitalizer):
A product to help revive the curl in permed hair that is growing out. It can also help reduce frizziness in a new perm.

Perm:
Many African-Americans call a relaxer a "perm."

Permanent Color:
Hair color that will grow out before it washes out, because it chemically changes the natural pigment of the hair.

pH:
The degree of acidity or alkalinity of any water-based solution. A pH of 7 is neutral, on a scale from 0 (very acidic) to 14 (very alkaline). Human hair seems to thrive best at 4.5 to 6.5—a slightly acidic pH level. Permanent hair coloring is an alkaline chemical process which temporarily raises the hair's pH to 10 or 11.

Photoaging:
Skin aging incurred through sun exposure.

Photosensitivity:
The "burning sensation" or heat that you can occasionally feel when nails are placed under a light during a manicure.

Pick:
A comb with widely spaced teeth. A pick is used more for "fluffing" a hairstyle than for actually combing or smoothing it.

Placentaisan Amino Acid:
A protein complex that replenishes moisture and protein in hair.

Pomade:
A type of hairdressing with the thickest consistency.

Porosity Equalizer:
A product used as "insurance" during a chemical service, to make sure the results will come out uniformly, even when some parts of the hair are more porous than others.

Porosity:
The hair's ability to absorb moisture. Hair must be slightly porous to allow conditioners and chemicals to ease their way into the hairshaft.

Post-Treatment:
A conditioner or normalizing lotion used immediately after a chemical service (hair color, perm relaxer) to close the cuticle.

Pre-Treatment:
A product applied to hair before a chemical service to make it more receptive to service or to condition hair.

Press(ing):
A term for thermal straightening.

Pressing Comb:
A thermal styling appliance which is pulled slowly through hair to straighten it.

Pressing Oil (Cream):
A waxy product that protects hair while it's being heat-styled, and that helps hold the hair's new shape.

Primer:
Substance that helps some acrylic nail extension products adhere better to the nail.

Processing Cap:
A lightweight, disposable plastic cap that holds in enough natural body heat for most perm products to work.

Processing Method:
How the waving lotion works on hair during the perming process is called "processing." Most perm products process at room temperature; some require heat from a dryer.

Processing Time:
The amount of time hair color, permanent waving solution or relaxer remains on the hair before being rinsed out.

Professional Formula:
A formulation designed especially for products used by salon professionals; some contain a higher concentration of certain ingredients.

Protein Treatment:
A treatment designed to rebuild strength in hair that has lost its elasticity by adding protein to the cortex.

Protein:
The substance from which hair is made. To strengthen damaged hair, some hair care products contain protein.

Ratt:
Hair foundations made of sponge-type material and used to create fullness or specific hairstyles, such as a chignon or French Twist.

Rearranger:
The first step in an ethnic curl service. This application of "thio" loosens the hair's natural curl, in preparation for the waving lotion.

Reconstructor:
A conditioner that adds internal and external protein to the hair.

Relax(ing):
To permanently straighten hair with chemicals.

Resins:
The ingredients in hairsprays and styling aids which give them holding power. There are two kinds of resins in beauty products: "holding" resins, to hold hair in place, and "memory" resins, to enable the hair to return to its

desired style, even after it is combed out or tousled.

Resistant:
A term for hair that is difficult to color, perm or relax, usually because it is not porous enough. The scales of the hair's cuticle lay too flat and tight against the hairshaft to allow chemicals to enter. Resistant hair must sometimes be pre-treated to get the cuticle to "open up" a bit.

Retin-A:
A vitamin-A derivative that acts as a topical anti-acne treatment.

Reverse Perm:
Takes curl out of hair.

Ridgefiller:
A type of basecoat which contains very fine grains of a material like talc. This material fills in ridges and small indentations in the natural nail to create a smoother surface for polishing.

Root Perm:
A perm service that is done on only the new growth of previously permed hair that has partially grown out.

"S" Pattern:
The well-defined "S" shape that a stylist looks for when checking a test curl in a perm.

Salicylic Acid:
Acts as a peeling agent and loosens debris in clogged pores. Present in many skin care products.

Scrubs or Exfoliating Products:
Scrubs, also called "exfoliants," loosen and remove the dead cells on the top layer of the skin, making the skin look smoother, finer and clearer. This process encourages and stimulates the formation of new skin cells. A washcloth, sloughing sponge, loofah or scrubbing product, such as washing grains, scrub

cleansers or sloughing cleansers, remove the excess oil that can clog pores and improve circulation, giving the skin a rosy glow. Exfoliating products are formulated for all skin types. However, do not over-scrub and irritate the skin. Use gentle circular motions and let the product do the work for you. Ingredients, such as alpha hydroxy acids, also work to exfoliate the skin without scrubbing.

Sculptured Nails:
Nail extensions made from acrylic or gels.

Sebum:
The natural oil that lubricates and protects the hair and scalp.

Semi-Permanent:
Hair color that gently penetrates the cortex without lifting the natural color and washes out gradually. No developer is needed, making this a non-oxidative type of color.

Setting Lotion:
Medium-hold products for hair that add volume, shape and style, and control curls.

Shape:
The term which refers to whether an individual hairshaft—or a full head of hair—is straight, wavy or very curly.

Sheen Spray:
The very lightest type of hairdressing.

Silicone:
Ingredient in some hair shiners that closes the hair cuticle and fills gaps where hair is broken.

Single Process:
Hair coloring that requires only one step to achieve the desired result.

Soap:
Basic toilet soaps combine an alkali with a fat, often a vegetable oil, and water. They are effective in cleaning grease, grime and

cosmetics, but can be drying or irritating to dry and sensitive skin types.

Soapless Cleansers:
Synthetic detergent liquids or bars that are less alkaline and richer lathering than basic soap. Non-soaps do not react with hard water to produce "soap scum" residue. Formulated for normal, dry or sensitive skin types.

SPF:
The acronym stands for "Sun Protection Factor."

Spiral Curls:
Long, corkscrew-shaped curls.

Spot Perm:
A permanent wave given on selected sections of hair instead of the entire head.

Spritz:
A spray-on styling aid. This term also describes the method of application—a light mist from a pump bottle. A spritz is different from a hairspray because it only holds a style—it doesn't "remember" it.

Stearyl Alcohol:
An ingredient of some conditioners and styling aids which smoothes and softens hair.

Streaking:
Applying color or bleach with a color brush, similar to painting.

Styling Gel:
A thick styling aid which is used for sculpting individual curls or "wet look" hairstyles.

Sunscreen (for nails):
A substance which absorbs the sun's ultraviolet (UV) light rays to prevent yellowing of the nails.

Superfatted Cleaners:
Basic soaps or detergents to which moisturizers such as cold cream, lanolin, olive oil or cocoa butter have been added. Superfatted

soaps generally contain between 5% and 15% fat as opposed to less than 2% in basic soap. Designed to both clean and moisturize normal-to-dry skin types. Often recommended for mature skin.

T-Zone:
The forehead, nose and chin.

Temporary Color:
A category of color products which wash out in one or two shampoos. They include rinses, mousses, hair color crayons and sprays.

Test Curl:
A strand of hair that is partially unwound from its perm rod to see how completely a perm has processed.

Texture:
The diameter (thickness) of the hairshaft, which determines how the hair "feels" (wiry, thin, etc.). There are three basic hair textures: coarse, medium and fine.

Texturizer:
A very mild relaxer product marketed for men.

Thermal Lotion:
A liquid styling aid formulated to protect hair from heat damage by hot rollers, blow dryers, curling irons, etc.

Thickener:
A styling aid which coats the hairshaft, causing it to stiffen and increase in diameter. Sometimes called a "texturizer."

Thio:
The term commonly used by stylists for ammonium thioglycolate (ATG), the key chemical ingredient in an alkaline perm. This is not an accurate expression because there are other, different types of "thio" chemicals (for example, glyceryl monothioglycolate, the key ingredient in acid perms).

Tint:
A permanent color which contains ammonia, so that it lightens the existing color and deposits new color in a single step.

Tip Overlay:
When a wrap or acrylic is applied over a nail tip to add strength and make it wear longer, the service is called a tip overlay.

Tips:
Pre-molded artificial fingernails, usually made of plastic, which are glued to natural nails.

Toluene:
An organic solvent used in nail polishes, topcoats and basecoats to help the polish stay on the nail.

Tone:
The indicator of how "warm" or "cool" a hair color is. Also referred to as the hair's "base color."

Toners (for skin):
Also called "fresheners" or "astringents," these products are generally used after cleansing to remove excess oil, cool and freshen the skin and temporarily tighten pores. There are two basic types: those that contain alcohol as a primary ingredient and those that do not. Alcohol helps dissolve dirt, oils and cosmetics but is also drying to the skin. Generally, fresheners and toners contain less alcohol than astringents, but they vary in alcohol content (as well as additional ingredients) from product to product. Alcohol-based products are not recommended for dry or sensitive skin. Alcohol-free toners often contain glycerin as well as botanical ingredients.

Topcoat:
A clear polish applied on top of color to add shine and protect the other coats of polish from chipping.

Transparent Soap:
Superfatted soap also containing a high glycerin content which is responsible for the soap's consistency and transparency. Effective for sensitive and normal-to-oily skin types. Glycerin is known as a humectant.

True-to-Rod-Size:
A perm product that creates curls the same size as the rods used.

Ultraviolet (UV) Light:
Can refer to light from the sun, or to lamps used in salons. UV light is used to "cure" (dry and harden) some nail gels.

UV Protectant:
Protects against ultraviolet (UV) rays.

Virgin Hair:
Hair that has not been previously permed, colored, straightened or otherwise chemically treated.

Viscosity:
The thickness of a liquid; its ability to flow. The higher the viscosity, the thicker the liquid.

Volumizing:
To make hair appear thicker.

Warm:
Refers to gold, orange or red-based tones in hair colors.

Washable Liquid Creams or Lotions:
These are basically soaps or detergents in a moisturizer base. Unlike cleansing creams, they are water soluble and can be rinsed with warm water. While formulated for different skin types, they are generally not recommended for oily skin.

Water Mold:
An infection which can grow under artificial—or even natural—nails. Water mold often turns the nail plate brown or greenish.

Wave Clamps:
Plastic or metal clamps used to hold wet hair in place to create waves while drying.

Waving Lotion:
The first chemical step in the perming process. The waving lotion penetrates into hair to disconnect the chemical bonds so the hair can be reshaped.

Weave:
A temporary way to add more hair to a person's head. Strands of human or synthetic hair are sewn or glued into place.

Weft:
A lock of synthetic or human hair used in bonding, weaving or on hair extensions.

Whiteheads:
A mixture of dead skin cells, oil and bacteria which produce bumps on the skin.

Working Spray:
A hairspray with the gentlest hold, typically used while hair is still being styled. Hair can be easily brushed after spraying with a working spray.

Wrap Cap:
A head covering, usually made of nylon or silk, worn to maintain the shape of a wrapped hairstyle. Also called a "doo rag."

Wrap:
A small piece of fabric (silk, linen or fiberglass) which is cut to the nail size and glued to a natural nail or nail tip, to add strength and/or length.

Wrapping Lotion:
Setting lotion used to create a tightly-molded, wrapped hairstyle.

Wrapping:
Rolling hair onto perm rods.

Index

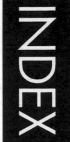

About The Editor

Beth Barrick-Hickey is national beauty advisor and a product development consultant to Sally Beauty Supply, the world's largest distributor of professional hair and nail care products. An 11-year veteran in the professional beauty industry, Ms. Barrick-Hickey is founder and president of Total Marketing Productions, a consulting and trade show production company. She is also co-owner of a leading professional nail product company in Arlington, Texas.

A licensed cosmetologist and former nail technician, Ms. Barrick-Hickey is well known in professional beauty circles for her education and training programs for professional nail technicians, beauty schools and professional beauty product distributors nationally and in Puerto Rico and Canada. She is a frequent guest on the LIFETIME cable television network program, "Our Home," and has appeared on "The Oprah Winfrey Show," "Mike & Maty" and "Joan Rivers" television talk shows.

The author of "New Business: How To Get It, How To Keep It" for salon professionals, Ms. Barrick-Hickey served on the board of the Nail Manufacturers Council, and is a member of the American Beauty Association (ABA), the Beauty and Barber Supply Institute (BBSI), and the National Cosmetology Association (NCA).

Prior to her professional beauty career, Ms. Barrick-Hickey was on-air talent for a cable television company where she helped develop and co-hosted a special beauty and fitness program.

References

1. "Panati's Extraordinary Origins of Everyday Things" by Charles Panati, 1987, Harper & Row Publishers.

2. "Why Did They Name It?" by Hannah Campbell, 1964, Fleet Press.

3. "Great American Brands and Topsellers" by David Powers Cleary, 1981, Fairchild.

4. "The Strange Story of False Hair" by John Woodforde, 1972, Drake.

5. "Accessories of Dress" by Katherine M. Lester and Bess V. Oerke, 1940, Manual Arts Press.

6. "400 Years Without A Comb" by Willie L. Morrow, 1984, Morrow's Marketing, Publishing, Research Development Corporation.

7. "Living Legends in Cosmetology" The Beginning by Carole Parks, Shoptalk, Jan./Feb., 1993.

8. "The New Medically Based No-Nonsense Beauty Book" by Deborah Chase, 1989, Avon Books.

9. Webster's Ninth New Collegiate Dictionary, 1986, Merriam-Webster.

10. "500 Beauty Solutions" by Beth Barrick-Hickey, 1994, Sourcebooks, Inc.

11. "Take Care of Your Skin" by Elaine Brumberg, 1989, Harper Perennial.

12. "Stage Makeup" by Richard Corson, 1975, Prentiss-Hall, Inc.

13. "Making Up by Rex: Beauty for Every Age, Every Woman" by Rex Hilverdink and Diana Lewis Jewell, 1986, Clarkson N. Potter, Inc.

14. "Super Skin: A Leading Dermatologist's Guide to the Latest Breakthroughs in Skin Care" by Nelson Lee Novick, 1988, Clarkson N. Potter, Inc.

15. "A Woman's Skin" by David M. Stoll, MD, 1994, Rutgers University Press.

16. "Aromatherapy for Woman: A Practical Guide to Essential Oils for Health and Beauty" by Maggie Tisserand, 1988, Healing Arts Press.

17. "The Art of Aromatherapy: The Healing and Beautifying Properties of the Essential Oils of Flowers and Herbs" by Robert B. Tisserand, 1977, Healing Arts Press.

18. "Cosmetics" Microsoft ® Encarta, Copyright © 1993 Microsoft Corporation. Copyright © 1993 Funk & Wagnall's Corporation. Bibliographic entries: B511, B612.

For product information and availability, call **1-800-284-7255**

We invite you to send us your beauty questions for inclusion in the next edition of *1001 Beauty Solutions*.
Address your questions to:

Attn: 1001 Beauty Solutions
The Hart Agency, Inc.
2811 McKinney Avenue, Suite 203
Dallas, TX 75204

Don't Miss These Other Great Titles From Sourcebooks!

Books for Women by Paula Peisner Coxe:

30 Days to a Sexier You
by Paula Peisner Coxe and Jessica Daniels

Introducing the 30-day attitude adjustment program for today's woman! *30 Days to a Sexier You* is designed to ignite the fire burning inside and bring out the uninhibited, sexy you.

ISBN: 1-57071-054-6; $6.95

"Paula Peisner Coxe is right on target! She knows what today's woman wants and needs."
—Allison Bell, Woman's World Magazine

Finding Time: Breathing Space for Women Who Do Too Much

For every woman too tired, too busy, or just too stressed to think of herself, this bestselling book shows you how to find or make time for yourself.

ISBN: 0-942061-33-0; $7.95

Finding Peace: Letting Go and Liking It
Reassess how to live your life, to contemplate, to forgive and accept. Learn the secrets of letting go and liking it.

ISBN: 1-57071-014-7; $7.95

Great Parenting Books by Sheila Ellison & Judith Gray!

365 Afterschool Activities: TV-Free Fun for Kids Ages 7-12

"Contains a wealth of engaging and fun-filled activities that are sure to keep kids playing, imagining and creating all year long."
—Brenda Pilson,
Creative Classroom Magazine
ISBN: 1-57071-080-5; $12.95

365 Days of Creative Play: For Children 2 Years & Up

"Activities that may work magic. Projects that you can do with your kids, and even better, activities they can do by themselves."
—Family Circle Magazine
ISBN: 1-57071-029-5; $12.95

365 Foods Kids Love to Eat: Fun, Nutritious and Kid-Tested

"A boon to busy parents and hungry kids alike."
—Parenting Magazine
ISBN: 1-57071-030-9; $12.95

For any of these books, or more copies of *1001 Beauty Solutions*, please contact your local bookseller, or call Sourcebooks at 708-961-3900. You may obtain a copy of our catalog by writing or faxing:

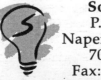

Sourcebooks
P.O. Box 372
Naperville, IL 60566
708-961-3900
Fax: 708-961-2168